Question Bank on
Veterinary Biochemistry

The Author

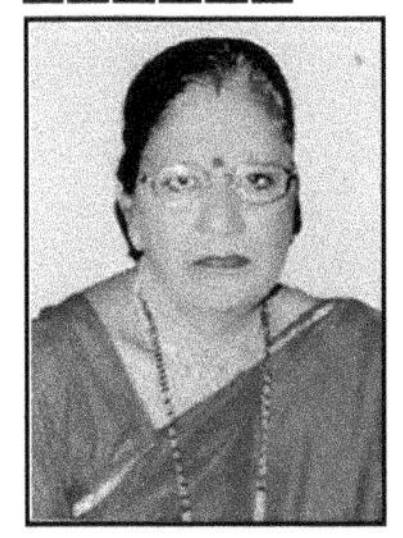

Dr. Neera Jain *M.Sc., Ph.D.* is Retired Associate Professor, Veterinary Biochemistry, College of Veterinary Science and Animal Husbandry, Nanaji Deshmukh Veterinary Science University, Jabalpur (M.P.).

She is also the recipient of a number of awards including the Professor Nils Lagerlof Memorial Medal' for Best Research Paper by Indian Veterinary Association, Chennai in 1998, Certificate of Honour from Central Poultry Diagnostic Laboratory, Jabalpur for establishing Diagnostic Laboratory and Honour of राष्ट्र भाषा गौरव की मानद उपाधि (2014) by Akhil Bhartiya Sevi Sansthan, Allahabad (U.P.) are at her credit. Besides this, she has published 4 books and various research papers in journals of repute.

Question Bank on *Veterinary Biochemistry*

For PG Entrance, JRF, SRF, ICAR-NET Ph.D Civil Services and other Competitive Exams

Dr Neera Jain

2018

Daya Publishing House®

A Division of

Astral International Pvt. Ltd.

New Delhi – 110 002

ISBN: 9789390384495 (Int. Edition)

Publisher's Note:

Every possible effort has been made to ensure that the information contained in this book is accurate at the time of going to press, and the publisher and author cannot accept responsibility for any errors or omissions, however caused. No responsibility for loss or damage occasioned to any person acting, or refraining from action, as a result of the material in this publication can be accepted by the editor, the publisher or the author. The Publisher is not associated with any product or vendor mentioned in the book. The contents of this work are intended to further general scientific research, understanding and discussion only. Readers should consult with a specialist where appropriate.

Every effort has been made to trace the owners of copyright material used in this book, if any. The author and the publisher will be grateful for any omission brought to their notice for acknowledgement in the future editions of the book.

Published by : **Daya Publishing House®**
A Division of
Astral International Pvt. Ltd.
– ISO 9001:2015 Certified Company –
4736/23, Ansari Road, Darya Ganj
New Delhi-110 002
Ph. 011-43549197, 23278134
E-mail: info@astralint.com
Website: www.astralint.com

Digitally Printed at : **Replika Press Pvt. Ltd.**

Preface

Biochemistry is the most fascinating subject, as it deals with language of life, be it human, animal, plant or micro-organism. No other science subject has as much applications as biochemistry to other disciplines of science. Since the students from other disciplines can not go deep in this subject, so the study in the form of question answer will definitely help them.

The book is so organized as to equip the readers with comprehensive knowledge of biochemistry and biotechnology.

Although I have made every efforts to make it error free. I welcome comments, criticism and suggestions from the faculty, students and other readers.

The book entitled "*Question Bank on Veterinary Biochemistry*" is an examination guide for the students. This book presents multiple choice questions along with answers key on various topics of Veterinary Biochemistry *viz.,* Carbohydrates, Lipids, Amino acids, Proteins, Vitamins, Hormones, Minerals etc. and Biotechnology. The idea of multiple choice questions will help to seek deep knowledge of subject concerned. In addition to this question bank will also be helpful/useful to Veterinary students at under-graduate, post-graduate and Ph.D. level. Not only the Veterinary students, but students from other faculty will also be benefitted. Above all, this the book will help in the preparation of competitive exams like ICAR-JRF, ICAR-SRF and ICAR NET. The book will also be useful for academic community.

Neera Jain

Contents

Abbreviations

Å: Armstrong
ABTS: Avidin biotin technique
ACTH: Adreno cortico tropic hormone
ADH: Antidiuretic hormone
ADP: Adenosine diphosphate
ALA: δ-amino levulinic acid
ALT: Alanine transaminase
AMP: Adenosine monophosphate
&: And
AST: Aspartate transaminase
ATP: Adenosine triphosphate
BMR: Basal metabolic rate
BUN: Blood urea nitrogen
cDNA: Complementary DNA
CDP: Cytidine diphosphate
CoA: Coenzyme A
Conc.: Concentration/concentrated
CSF: Cerebrospinal fluid
Da: Dalton
DAB: Diaminobenzidine

°C: Degree centigrade
DFP: Di-isopropyl fluorophosphate
DIA: Dot Immunobinding assay
dl: Decilitre
DNA: Deoxyribonucleic acid
DNAse: Deoxyribo nuclease
EDTA: Ethylene diamine tetraacetic acid
EIA: Enzyme immuno assay
ELISA: Enzyme linked immunosorbent assay
ESR: Erythrocyte sedimentation rate
FAD: Flavin adenine dinucleotide
FADP: Flavin adenine dinucleotide phosphate
FDP: Fructose 1, 6-diphosphate
FIGLU: Formimino glutamate
FITC: Fluorescein isothiocyanate
FMN: Flavin mononucleotide
FRET: Flourescence resonance energy transfer
FSH: Follice stimulating hormone
GDP: Guanosine diphosphate
g: Gram
HbS: Sickle cell hemoglobin
HbA: Adult hemoglobin
HCG: Human chorionic gonadotropin
HDL: High density lipoprotein
HIV: Human immunodeficiency virus
HGPRT: Hypoxanthine guanine phosphoribosyl transferase
HPLC: High pressure liquid chromatography
Hrs: Hours
Ig: Immunoglobulin
ITP: Ionosine triphosphate
IU: International Unit
L: Litre
LDL: Low density lipoprotein
mRNA: Messenger RNA

µm: Micro meter
M: Molarity
µg: Microgram
mg: Miligram
ml: Mililitre
mµ: Milimicron
mmole: Milimole
Min: Minute
ml: Mililitre
MOET: Multiple ovulation with embryo transfer
N: Normality
NAD: Nicotinamide adenine dinucleotide
NADP: Nicotinamide adenine dinucleotide phosphate
NADPH: Reduced nicotinamide adenine dinucleotide phosphate
NMR: Nuclear Magnetic resonance
nm: nanometer
No.: Number
OPD: Orthophenylene diamine dihydrochloride
PAGE: Polyacrylamide gel electrophoresis
PBG: Porphobilinogen
PBS: Phosphate buffer saline
PCR: Polymerase chain reaction
PFK: Phosphofructokinase
PLP: Pyridoxal phosphate
pmol: Picomol
PRPP: Pyrophosphoribosyl-5-phosphate
RBC: Red blood corpuscles
RIA: Radioimmuno assay
rRNA: Ribosomal RNA
RNAse: Ribonuclease
SDS: Starch dodecyl sulphate
Sec: Second
SnRNA: Small nuclear ribonucleic acid
T: Titre

TCA: Tricarboxylic acid
TPN: Triphosphopyridine nucleotide
TPP: Thiamine pyrophosphate
tRNA: Transfer RNA
UDP: Uridine diphosphate
UDPG: Uridine diphosphate glucose
UV: Ultraviolet
VFA: Volatile fatty acid
VLDL: Very low density lipoprotein

Chapter 1

Biophysical Chemistry

1. **Which one is the heaviest particulate component of the cell?**
   (a) Nucleus (b) Mitochondria
   (c) Cytoplasm (d) Golgi apparatus

2. **Which one is the largest particulate of the cytoplasm?**
   (a) Lysosomes (b) Mitochondria
   (c) Golgi apparatus (d) Endoplasmic reticulum

3. **Which particulate component of the cell is considered as power house of the cell?**
   (a) Nucleus (b) Cell membrane
   (c) Mitochondria (d) Golgi apparatus

4. **The degradative processes are categorized under the heading of:**
   (a) Anabolism (b) Catabolism
   (c) Metabolism (d) None of them

5. **The exchange of material takes place:**
   (a) Only by diffusion (b) Only by active transport
   (c) Only by pinocytosis (d) All of them

6. **Which one is the strongest intermolecular force?**
   (a) Hydrogen bond (b) Dipole-dipole
   (c) Vanderwaal's forces (d) All are equal

7. **The pH value of an acidic solution will be:**
   (a) 7 (b) More than 7
   (c) Less than 7 (d) None of them

8. **The pH value of blood is 7.4. The buffer system, which helps in maintaining it, consists of:**
   (a) CH_3COOH–CH_3COONa (b) H_2CO_3- $NaHCO_3$
   (c) Glycine + HCl (d) Protein buffers

9. **pH of water at 22°C is 7.0, its value at 38°C will be:**
   (a) 7.0 (b) 10.23
   (c) 6.74 (d) Not definite

10. **The difference in pH between arterial and venous blood is rarely more than:**
    (a) 0.02 (b) 0.03
    (c) 0.04 (d) 0.06

11. **The average pH of urine is:**
    (a) 7.0 (b) 6.0
    (c) 8.0 (d) 0.0

12. **The pH of blood is 7.4, then the ratio between of H_2CO_3 and $NaHCO_3$ is:**
    (a) 1:10 (b) 1:20
    (c) 1:25 (d) 1:30

13. **The phenomenon of osmosis is opposite to that of:**
    (a) Diffusion (b) Effusion
    (c) Affusion (d) Coagulation

14. **If a cell is immersed in a concentrated solution, it follows the phenomenon of:**
    (a) Plasmolysis (b) Plasmoptysis
    (c) Either of the two (d) None of them

15. **The purgative action of epson salt follows which phenomenon:**
    (a) Absorption (b) Adsorption
    (c) Diffusion (d) Osmosis

16. **The surface tension of a solution is increased by:**
    (a) Bile salts (b) Bile acids
    (c) Conc. H_2SO_4 (d) Acetic acid

17. Surface tension is lowered by:

(a) Ammonia
(b) Sodium hydroxide
(c) Potassium hydroxide
(d) Aluminium hydroxide

18. Adsorption is applied in the purification of:

(a) Vitamins
(b) Hormones
(c) Enzymes
(d) Co-enzymes

19. Bile salts make emulsification with fat for the action of:

(a) Pepsin
(b) Lipase
(c) Amylase
(d) Trypsin

20. Fatty acids can be transported into and out of the mitochondria through:

(a) Active transport
(b) Facilitated transfer
(c) Non-facilitated transfer
(d) None of them

21. The absorption of intact protein from the gut in new born babies takes place by:

(a) Active transport
(b) Diffusion
(c) Pinocytosis
(d) None of them

22. Thyroid function is determined by:

(a) Na^{24}
(b) Co^{60}
(c) I^{131}
(d) Fe^{59}

23. Na^{24} is used for diagnosis of:

(a) Brain tumors
(b) Pernicious anemia
(c) Thyroid function
(d) Arterial diseases

24. Study of protein biosynthesis involves the use of:

(a) Na^{24}
(b) N^{15}
(c) Ca^{45}
(d) Co^{60}

25. Each water molecule is surrounded by number of water molecules by hydrogen bond:

(a) 4
(b) 5
(c) 6
(d) 8

26. During severe muscular exercise, when the blood lactic acid content rises over 100mg per 100ml, the pH of blood:

(a) Slightly increases
(b) Highly increases
(c) Slightly decreases
(d) Markedly decreases

27. The osmotic pressure of a solution increases with the rise in:

(a) Temperature (b) Cold

(c) Humidity (d) Rancidity

28. The intracellular fluid of red cells and the red cell membrane in 0.92% NaCl solution maintains a relation:

(a) Hypertonic (b) Hypotonic

(c) Isotonic (d) None of them

29. Hemolysis is caused by the dilution of RBC by:

(a) Diffusion (b) Osmosis

(c) Effusion (d) Imbibation

30. Adsorption decreases with the rise in:

(a) Cold (b) Humidity

(c) Dryness (d) Temperature

31. The following is the hydrotropic substance:

(a) Hydrochloric acid (b) Nitric acid

(c) Hippuric acid (d) Salicylic acid

32. Pernicious anemia is diagnosed by the radioactive substance:

(a) Cl^{36} (b) P^{32}

(c) Co^{60} (d) Fe^{59}

33. Some of the calcium phosphate of the blood is held in colloidal suspension by the protective action of:

(a) Lipids (b) Carbohydrates

(c) Proteins (d) Minerals

34. The serum colloidal protein particles may be precipitated by the addition of large amount of:

(a) Calcium sulphate (b) Ammonium sulphate

(c) Barium sulphate (d) Magnesium sulphate

35. The size of each colloidal particle in nm is:

(a) 4 to 40 (b) 6 to 60

(c) 8 to 80 (d) 10 to 100

36. The viscosity of a liquid increases due to the presence of:

(a) Suspended particles (b) Soluble particles

(c) Small sized particles (d) None of them

37. Lyophilic colloids undergo:

(a) Irreversible coagulation
(b) Reversible coagulation
(c) Both (a) and (b)
(d) None of them

38. Lyophobic colloids undergo:

(a) Irreversible coagulation
(b) Reversible coagulation
(c) Both (a) and (b)
(d) None of them

39. Na^+ and K^+ transport occur through:

(a) α-sub-unit
(b) β-sub-unit
(c) γ-sub-unit
(d) None of them

40. The atoms having the same atomic number but different atomic weights are said to be:

(a) Isotopes
(b) Isobars
(c) Both (a) and (b)
(d) None of them

41. The force with which surface molecules are held together is called:

(a) Surface tension
(b) Osmosis
(c) Viscosity
(d) None of them

42. The resistance experienced by one layer of a liquid in moving over the other is called:

(a) Viscosity
(b) surface tension
(c) Osmosis
(d) None of them

43. Temperature can not alter the pH of a solution of:

(a) 0.1N HCl
(b) 0.2N HCl
(c) 0.3N HCl
(d) None of them

44. The transport of most ions as compared to non-electrolytes occur:

(a) Slowly
(b) Fast
(c) Same speed
(d) None of them

45. With a rise in temperature, the adsorption:

(a) Increases
(b) Decreases
(c) Remains same
(d) None of them

46. The buffering system are similar for:

(a) Lymph
(b) Blood
(c) Cerebrospinal fluid
(d) All of them

47. Acidosis is of the type:

(a) Respiratory (b) Metabolic
(c) Both (a) and (b) (d) None of them

48. Some of the carrier proteins are called:

(a) Uniports (b) Symports
(c) Both (a) and (b) (d) None of them

49. An emulsoid may be changed into a suspensoid by:

(a) Dehydration (b) Hydrolysis
(c) Both (a) and (b) (d) None of them

50. Osmotic pressure of the soaps is:

(a) Lower (b) Higher
(c) Both (a) and (b) (d) None of them

51. Water is not expelled by squeezing in:

(a) Imbibition (b) Precipitation
(c) Combination (d) Dilution

52. Lipids and proteins which are both effective in lowering surface tension are found concentrated in the cell wall following the principle of:

(a) Johnson-John (b) Gibbs Thomson
(c) Peterson-Pollen (d) None of them

53. In simple diffusion ds/dt (C_0-C_1) can be expressed by the modification of:

(a) Rongent's Law (b) Fabry's Law
(c) Pollinger's Law (d) Fick's Law

54. The pH of gastric juice of infants:

(a) 2.0 (b) 4.0
(c) 4.5 (d) 5.0

55. The pH of water is 7.0 at the temperature in centigrade:

(a) 22 (b) 30
(c) 37 (d) 40

56. The pH of buffer is determined by pH = Pka + log [salt/acid] which is also known as the equation of:

(a) Henderson – Joules (b) Henderson – Smith
(c) Henderson – Harris (d) Henderson Hasselbalch

57. In case of non-homogenous solution, diffusion is expressed as: ds/dt = DA dc/dx by:

(a) Fick's Law
(b) Petersons' Law
(c) Faraday's Law
(d) Dick's Law

58. The osmotic pressure of a solution relating to the solute molecules depends on the:

(a) Size
(b) Shape
(c) Number
(d) Volume

59. The spreading of solute molecules throughout the water molecules is known as:

(a) Diffusion
(b) Dispersion
(c) Adsorption
(d) None of them

60. Surface tension is involved in the process of:

(a) Digestion
(b) Absorption
(c) Respiration
(d) None of them

61. Number of gram equivalent of solute in 1L is known as:

(a) Normality
(b) Molarity
(c) Molality
(d) None of them

62. Number of moles of solute per 100g of solvent is known as:

(a) Molality
(b) Normality
(c) Molarity
(d) None of them

63. Number of grams of dissolved substance contained in 1ml of solution is known as:

(a) Titre
(b) Standard solution
(c) Normal solution
(d) None of them

64. Number of parts of the substance in one million parts of solution is known as:

(a) Percent concentration
(b) Parts per million
(c) Titre
(d) None of them

65. For the acid base titration, indicator used is:

(a) Methyl red
(b) Methyl orange
(c) Phenolphthalein
(d) (a) or (b) or (c)

66. Indicators possess different colour in:

(a) Dissociated form (b) Undissociated form

(c) Both (a) and (b) (d) None of them

67. Normality of concentrated hydrochloric acid is:

(a) 16 N (b) 36 N

(c) 12 N (d) None of them

68. Concentrated sulphuric acid's normality is:

(a) 16 N (b) 12 N

(c) 36 N (d) None of them

69. Normality of concentrated nitric acid is:

(a) 16 N (b) 36 N

(c) 12 N (d) None of them

70. For preparing N/10 H_2SO_4 in 1000ml, volume of H_2SO_4 required will be:

(a) 2.8ml (b) 3.6ml

(c) 5.0ml (d) 5.6ml

71. Volume of HCl required for preparing 1N HCl in 1 litre will be:

(a) 82ml (b) 28ml

(c) 63ml (d) None of them

72. Volume of HNO_3 required for preparing 0.1 N HNO_3 in 500ml will be:

(a) 3.15ml (b) 4.25ml

(c) 5.25ml (d) 6.25ml

73. The substances accepting electron are:

(a) Oxidizing agents (b) Reducing agents

(c) Either (a) or (b) (d) Neither (a) or (b)

74. The substances oxidized to higher valency state, but reduce other substances are:

(a) Reducing agents (b) Oxidizing agents

(c) Either (a) or (b) (d) Neither (a) or (b)

75. Diffusion of solvent is due to the motion of:

(a) Solute molecule from a concentrated solution into solvent

(b) Solvent molecule into concentrated solution

(c) Both (a) and (b)

(d) None of them

76. Equivalent weight of $KMnO_4$ in acid medium is:

(a) 158
(b) 31.6
(c) 63
(d) None of them

77. Equivalent weight of $KMnO_4$ in alkaline medium is:

(a) 31.6
(b) 158
(c) 63
(d) None of them

78. Molarity is denoted by:

(a) N
(b) M
(c) T
(d) None of them

79. Acid base titration is used for the quantitative determination of:

(a) Acid
(b) Base
(c) Salt
(d) Both (a) and (b)

80. Oxidation reduction titration is used for the quantitative determination of:

(a) Oxidizing agent
(b) Reducing agent
(c) Both (a) and (b)
(d) None of them

Answer Key

1	(a)	21	(c)	41	(a)	61	(a)
2	(b)	22	(c)	42	(a)	62	(a)
3	(c)	23	(d)	43	(a)	63	(a)
4	(b)	24	(b)	44	(a)	64	(b)
5	(d)	25	(a)	45	(b)	65	(d)
6	(a)	26	(d)	46	(d)	66	(c)
7	(c)	27	(a)	47	(c)	67	(c)
8	(b)	28	(c)	48	(c)	68	(c)
9	(c)	29	(b)	49	(a)	69	(a)
10	(c)	30	(d)	50	(a)	70	(a)
11	(b)	31	(c)	51	(a)	71	(a)
12	(b)	32	(c)	52	(b)	72	(a)
13	(a)	33	(c)	53	(d)	73	(a)
14	(a)	34	(b)	54	(a)	74	(a)
15	(d)	35	(d)	55	(a)	75	(c)
16	(c)	36	(a)	56	(d)	76	(b)
17	(c)	37	(b)	57	(a)	77	(b)
18	(c)	38	(a)	58	(c)	78	(b)
19	(b)	39	(a)	59	(a)	79	(d)
20	(b)	40	(a)	60	(a)	80	(c)

Chapter 2

Carbohydrates and their Metabolism

1. **Various glucose units in glycogen are linked by:**
   (a) 1,4-linkage
   (b) 1,6-linkage
   (c) Both of the linkages
   (d) None of the above linkages
2. **Possible number of isomers of glucose is:**
   (a) 4
   (b) 8
   (c) 12
   (d) 16
3. **Which one of the following is epimer of glucose?**
   (a) Fructose
   (b) Ribose
   (c) Galactose
   (d) Cellulose
4. **Cellulose is made of molecules of:**
   (a) α-glucose
   (b) β-glucose
   (c) Both (a) and (b)
   (d) None of the them
5. **Honey contains the hydrolytic product of:**
   (a) Lactose
   (b) Maltose
   (c) Starch
   (d) Inulin

6. **Which of the following compound is found to be present in heart valves?**
   (a) Hyaluronic acid
   (b) Chondroitin sulphate
   (c) Heparin
   (d) Glucosamine

7. **Which of the monosaccharide has maximum rate of absorption in small intestine?**
   (a) Galactose
   (b) Glucose
   (c) Fructose
   (d) Mannose

8. **Glycosides are compounds formed by monosaccharides with alcohol. Which carbon atom of monosaccharides reacts in this reaction?**
   (a) C_1
   (b) C_4
   (c) C_5
   (d) C_6

9. **The carbon atoms involved in osazone formation:**
   (a) 1 and 2
   (b) 2 and 3
   (c) 3 and 4
   (d) 5 and 6

10. **α-D glucopyranose molecule contains number of asymmetric c-atoms:**
    (a) 5
    (b) 2
    (c) 3
    (d) 4

11. **Ribose and Deoxyribose differ in structure around c-atom:**
    (a) 2
    (b) 3
    (c) 4
    (d) 5

12. **Sorbitol and mannitol are obtained by the reduction of :**
    (a) Glucose
    (b) Fructose
    (c) Mannose
    (d) None of them

13. **Naturally occurring glucose belongs to:**
    (a) D-series
    (b) L-series
    (c) Both (a) and (b)
    (d) None of them

14. **Glucuronic acid is formed by the oxidation of glucose at:**
    (a) 6th c-atom
    (b) 2nd c-atom
    (c) 4th c-atom
    (d) All of them

15. **Heparin is an:**
    (a) Anticoagulant
    (b) Antioxidant
    (c) Both (a) and (b)
    (d) None of them

16. Sucrose is:

(a) Reducing sugar (b) Non-reducing sugar
(c) Both (a) and (b) (d) None of them

17. Glucose and galactose are obtained by the hydrolysis of:

(a) Maltose (b) Lactose
(c) Sucrose (d) All of them

18. Ketohexoses have number of asymmetric c-atoms:

(a) 1 (b) 2
(c) 3 (d) 4

19. The term pyranose and furanose are derived from:

(a) Pyran (b) Furan
(c) Pyran and Furan (d) None of them

20. Anomers are the compounds which differ in configuration only at:

(a) C_1 (b) C_2
(c) C_3 (d) C_4

21. Mucopolysaccharides are:

(a) Homopolysaccharides (b) Heteropolysaccharides
(c) Both (a) and (b) (d) None of them

22. The glycosidic bond at the branching points in the structure of starch is:

(a) α-1, 4- glycosidic bond (b) α-1, 6- glycosidic bond
(c) Both (a) and (b) (d) None of them

23. Which of the following sugars is a tetrose?

(a) Galactose (b) Fructose
(c) Idose (d) Erythrose

24. Alcohol dehydrogenase from liver contains:

(a) Sodium (b) Potassium
(c) Copper (d) Zinc

25. NADP-linked dehydrogenases in extramitochondria are found to synthesize:

(a) Carbohydrates (b) Fatty acids
(c) Vitamins (d) Urea

26. The uncoupling agent of oxidative phosphorylation is:

(a) Barbiturates (b) Penicillin

(c) Antimycin (d) Dicoumarol

27. When substrates are oxidized through a NAD-linked dehydrogenase, the P:O ratio is:

(a) 1 (b) 2

(c) 3 (d) 4

28. Which one of the following is not a monosaccharide?

(a) Glucose (b) Fructose

(c) Galactose (d) Lactose

29. Which one of the following is not a disaccharide?

(a) Sucrose (b) Maltose

(c) Lactose (d) Starch

30. Phosphorylase a in muscle in a tetramer containing 4 molecules of:

(a) ATP (b) NAD^+

(c) Pyridoxal phosphate (d) CoA

31. Barfoed's solution is not reduced by:

(a) Glucose (b) Sucrose

(c) Mannose (d) Ribose

32. Glycogen is a polysaccharide made up of infinite number of glucose units linked with each other:

(a) Only by 1,4-linkage (b) Only by 1, 6-linkage

(c) By both types of linkages (d) None of the above type

33. Which of the following sugar is found in RNA?

(a) Xylose (b) Threose

(c) Ribose (d) Glucose

34. Which of the following is a sugar alcohol?

(a) Gluconic acid (b) Maltose

(c) Mannitol (d) None of them

35. Glucose can not be classified as:

(a) Hexose (b) Oligosaccharide

(c) Monosaccharide (d) Aldose

36. Red colour with iodine solution is given by:

(a) Glycogen (b) Starch

(c) Dextrin (d) None of them

37. Which one of the following does not reduce Fehling solution?

(a) Glucose (b) Fructose

(c) Sucrose (d) Lactose

38. Glucose absorption may be decreased in:

(a) Oedema (b) Nephritis

(c) Rickets (d) Osteomyelitis

39. Benedict reagent is not reduced by:

(a) Glucose (b) Galactose

(c) Fructose (d) Sucrose

40. Iodine solution gives no colour with :

(a) Cellulose (b) Starch

(c) Glycogen (d) Dextrin

41. When D-ribose is dehydrated with concentrated H_2SO_4, it yields:

(a) D-ribitol (b) Furfural

(c) Ribonic acid (d) None of them

42. Synthesis of 2,3-biphosphoglycerate occurs in tissues mainly:

(a) Liver (b) Kidney

(c) Erythrocytes (d) Brain

43. One of the following enzymes in glycolysis catalyses an irreversible reaction:

(a) Hexokinase (b) Phosphofructokinase

(c) Pyruvate kinase (d) All of them

44. The number of ATP produced when a molecule of acetyl CoA is oxidized through citric acid cycle:

(a) 12 (b) 24

(c) 38 (d) 15

45. The common currency of energy in biological reaction is:

(a) AMP (b) ADP

(c) ATP (d) UDPG

46. In Kreb cycle, which step involves substrate level phosphorylation:

(a) Conversion of oxalosuccinate to α-ketoglutarate

(b) Conversion of α-ketoglutarate to succinyl CoA

(c) Conversion of succinyl CoA to succinate

(d) Conversion of succinate to fumarate

47. Which of the following is not a polymer of glucose?

(a) Amylose (b) Cellulose

(c) Inulin (d) Glycogen

48. Oxidation of aldehyde group (C_1) of glucose results in the formation of:

(a) Glucuronic acid (b) Mucic acid

(c) Gluconic acid (d) None of them

49. Reduction of glucose with calcium in water produces:

(a) Sorbitol (b) Dulcitol

(c) Mannitol (d) None of them

50. The repeating disaccharide unit in cellulose is:

(a) Dextrin (b) Maltose

(c) Cellobiose (d) Dextrose

51. The reducing ability of carbohydrate is due to the presence of/ formation of:

(a) A free carboxyl group (b) A free hydroxyl group

(c) Enediol formation (d) Presence of α-1,4 linkage

52. Reactions between a hemiacetal group to another-OH group yields:

(a) Peptide bond (b) Glycosidic bond

(c) Phosphodiester bond (d) None of them

53. Conversion of citrate to isocitrate is catalysed by:

(a) Citrate (b) Isocitrase

(c) Aconitase (d) Carboxylase

54. Muscular glycogen does not directly contribute to blood glucose due to:

(a) Absence of fructose-6-phosphatase

(b) Absence of glucose-6-phosphatase

(c) Both (a) and (b)

(d) None of them

55. Which of the following enzymes in glycolytic pathway is inhibited by fluoride?

(a) Glyceraldehyde 3-P-dehydrogenase (b) Phosphoglycerate kinase

(c) Pyruvate kinase (d) Enolase

56. Dehydrogenases involved in HMP shunt are specific for:

(a) NADPH (b) NAD^+

(c) FAD (d) None of them

57. The number of ATP produced when one free glucose molecule undergoes glycolysis under aerobic condition:

(a) 2 (b) 12

(c) 8 (d) 38

58. Gluconeogenesis is repressed by:

(a) Insulin (b) Glucocorticoid

(c) AMP (d) ADP

59. Acetyl CoA carboxylase promoted by:

(a) Citrate (b) Palmitoyl CoA

(c) NADPH (d) NADP

60. Urine of a patient suffering from diabetic coma has:

(a) Glucose (b) Ketone bodies

(c) Both (a) and (b) (d) None of them

61. In juvenile diabetes which pancreatic cells are exhausted:

(a) α-cells (b) β-cells

(c) Both (a) and (b) (d) None of them

62. Insulin is destroyed by:

(a) Insulinase (b) Peptidase

(c) Both (a) and (b) (d) None of them

63. During anger, anxiety and fear, blood sugar level:

(a) Increases (b) Decreases

(c) Remains same (d) None of them

64. Gluconeogenesis mainly takes place in:

(a) Liver (b) Kidney

(c) Both (a) and (b) (d) None of them

65. The reduced NAD^+ enters the respiratory chain and the number of ATP produced is:

(a) 1 (b) 2
(c) 3 (d) 4

66. Uronic acid functions as:

(a) Structural material (b) Detoxicating agent
(c) Both (a) and (b) (d) None of them

67. Carbohydrates are digested mainly in:

(a) Small intestine (b) Large intestine
(c) Both (a) and (b) (d) None of them

68. Main site of glycolysis is:

(a) Brain (b) Spleen
(c) Muscles (d) Kidney

69. Enzymes of TCA cycle are found in:

(a) Cytoplasm (b) Endoplasmic reticulum
(c) Lysosomes (d) Mitochondria

70. The most abundantly phosphate ester found in erythrocytes is:

(a) Glucose-6-phosphate (b) Fructose-6-phosphate
(c) Fructose 1,6-diphosphate (d) 2,3-diphosphoglycerate

71. Activator for gluconeogenesis is:

(a) Acetyl CoA (b) Citrate
(c) FDP (d) NADP

72. Effector hormone for lipogenesis is:

(a) Insulin (b) Glucocorticoid
(c) Thyroxine (d) Vasopressin

73. Inhibitor for glycolysis is:

(a) Citrate (b) NADPH
(c) Phosphorylase (d) ADP

74. Cell cycle has phase in number:

(a) 1 (b) 2
(c) 3 (d) 4

75. Major regulatory enzyme for TCA cycle is:

(a) Citrate synthase (b) Phosphorylase

(c) Glucose-6-phosphate dehydrogenase (d) Glycogen synthase

76. Inhibitor for TCA cycle is:

(a) ATP (b) Citrate

(c) ADP (d) AMP

77. Pentose phosphate pathway is induced by:

(a) Insulin (b) Epinephrine

(c) Glucagon (d) Citrate

78. D-galactose differ from D-glucose in orientation of H and OH on carbon atom:

(a) 2 (b) 3

(c) 4 (d) 5

79. The compound implicated in the development of cataract in diabetic patient is:

(a) Sorbitol (b) Dulcitol

(c) Mannitol (d) None of them

80. In normal resting state, most of the blood glucose burned as fuel is consumed by:

(a) Liver (b) Kidney

(c) Brain (d) Adipose tissue

81. Which of the following metabolic pathway is most correctly considered as amphibolic?

(a) Lipolysis (b) Glycolysis

(c) Citric acid cycle (d) Gluconeogenesis

82. Glycogenolysis can only be effective, if the level of cAMP is:

(a) Increased (b) Decreased

(c) Remain static (d) None of them

83. Which of the following intermediates of metabolism cannot be a precursor of glucose?

(a) Lactate (b) Pyruvate

(c) Alanine (d) Acetyl CoA

84. The main product of glycolysis in skeletal muscles under aerobic condition is:

(a) Pyruvic acid (b) Lactic acid
(c) Both (a) and (b) (d) None of them

85. Glycogenolysis in muscles produces:

(a) Glucose (b) Pyruvate
(c) Lactate (d) Glucose-6-phosphate

86. Glycogenesis is a process in which glycogen is synthesized from:

(a) Glucose (b) Pyruvate
(c) Lactate (d) Propionic acid

87. Each branch of amylopectin is at an interval of glucose units:

(a) 14-20 (b) 24-30
(c) 34-40 (d) 44-50

88. Glycogen synthetase activity is depressed by:

(a) Glucose (b) Insulin
(c) Cyclic AMP (d) Fructokinase

89. The absorption of glucose is interfered by the deficiency of:

(a) Vitamin A (b) Thiamine
(c) Magnesium sulphate (d) Ferrous sulphate

90. Human heart muscle contains:

(a) D-ribose (b) D-lyxose
(c) D-xylose (d) D-Arabinose

91. Racemic mixtures are:

(a) Optically active (b) Optically inactive
(c) Either (a) or (b) (d) Neither (a) or (b)

92. The branching enzyme acts on the glycogen when the main chain is lengthened by:

(a) 1-6 glucose units (b) 2-7 glucose units
(c) 3-9 glucose units (d) 6-11 glucose units

93. The term dextrorotatory (+) used for the compounds which rotate the plane of polarized light to:

(a) Right (b) Left
(c) Either (a) or (b) (d) None of them

94. The main product of glycolysis in skeletal muscles (under anaerobic condition) is:

(a) Pyruvate (b) Lactate

(c) Both (a) and (b) (d) None of them

95. The main product of glycolysis under aerobic condition is:

(a) Pyruvate (b) Lactate

(c) Both (a) and (b) (d) None of them

96. The net number of moles of ATP produced when one glycosyl unit of glycogen undergoes glycolysis under anaerobic condition is:

(a) 1 (b) 2

(c) 3 (d) 4

97. Glucose is removed from the blood following a meal by:

(a) Hexokinase (b) Glucokinase

(c) Both (a) and (b) (d) None of them

98. Pyruvate is accumulated by the dietary deficiency of:

(a) Vitamin B_1 (b) Vitamin B_2

(c) Vitamin B_6 (d) Vitamin B_{12}

99. The enzyme pyruvate dehydrogenase is found to be a complex system of different enzymes. The approximate total no. of moles of the various enzymes in one mole of this enzyme is:

(a) 19 (b) 29

(c) 38 (d) 49

100. Carbohydrates are the organic compounds made up of:

(a) Carbon (b) Hydrogen

(c) Oxygen (d) All of them

101. Hexokinase has a high affinity for glucose than:

(a) Fructokinase (b) Galactokinase

(c) Glucokinase (d) All of them

102. Conversion of fructose 1, 6-diphosphate to fructose-6-phosphate is stimulated by:

(a) Glucagon (b) Insulin

(c) ACTH (d) None of them

103. Activation of the inactive phosphorylase is stimulated by:

(a) ATP
(b) NAD^+
(c) Cyclic AMP
(d) None of them

104. Cyclic AMP is formed from ATP by the enzyme adenylate cyclase which is activated by the hormone:

(a) Insulin
(b) Epinephrine
(c) Testosterone
(d) Progesterone

105. The synthesis of adenylate cyclase is increased by:

(a) Thyroid hormones
(b) Growth hormones
(c) ACTH
(d) FSH

106. Dihydroxyacetonephosphate and glyceraldehydes 3-phosphate are inter converted by:

(a) Dihydroxy acetone phosphorylase
(b) Triose isomerase
(c) Phosphotriose isomerase
(d) Diphosphotriose isomerase

107. In HMP shunt, 6-phosphogluconate is oxidized to 3-keto-6 phosphogluconate in presence of:

(a) NAD^+
(b) $NADP^+$
(c) FAD^+
(d) $FADP^+$

108. In liver fructokinase converts fructose to:

(a) Fructose-1-phosphate
(b) Fructose-6-phosphate
(c) Fructose-1, 6 diphosphate
(d) Glucose-1-phosphate

109. Lactose is formed in mammary gland under the influence of lactose synthetase by the reaction of:

(a) Glucose and galactose
(b) UDP-glucose and galactose
(c) UDP-galactose and glucose
(d) UDP glucose and UDP-galactose

110. Mucopolysaccharides consist of repeating of disaccharide molecules consisting of:

(a) Two monosaccharides
(b) Glucuronic acid + amino sugar
(c) Uronic acid + acetylated amino sugar
(d) None of them

111. Which of the following is not a mucopolysaccharide?

(a) Heparin (b) Chondroitin sulphate

(c) Sialic acid (d) Insulin

112. In case of insufficient supply of glucose gluconeogenesis is the important source of glucose in:

(a) Muscles (b) Adipose tissue

(c) Nervous tissue (d) Liver

113. Function of brain is disturbed when blood glucose level falls from the normal fasting value (80mg/100ml) to:

(a) 60mg/100ml (b) 40mg/100ml

(c) 20mg/100ml (d) 10mg/100ml

114. Which of the hormone decreases blood sugar level?

(a) Glucagon (b) Epinephrine

(c) Glucocorticoids (d) Insulin

115. The renal threshold value for glucose is:

(a) 80mg/100ml (b) 120mg/100ml

(c) 180mg/100ml (d) 200mg/100ml

116. Amount of sugar in urine of a normal individual is:

(a) 0.05% (b) 0.5%

(c) 1% (d) > 1%

117. Diabetes mellitus is characterized by:

(a) Glycosuria (b) Polyuria

(c) Polydipsia (d) All the three

118. Insulin is given in the form of:

(a) In water (b) In alcohol

(c) In tissue fluid (d) Protamine Zinc Insulin

119. Fructose 1-phosphate is splitted into glyceraldehyde and di-hydroxy acetone phosphate by the enzyme:

(a) Enolase (b) Aldolase A

(c) Aldolase B (d) Aldolase A and B

120. Glucose-6-phosphatase is absent from:

(a) Intestine (b) Kidney

(c) Heart (d) Adipose tissue

121. Fructokinase is present in:

(a) Intestine
(b) Brain
(c) Heart
(d) Adipose tissue

122. Steps leading to decomposition of pyruvate via oxalate to carbon dioxide are known as:

(a) Kreb cycle
(b) Citric acid cycle
(c) TCA cycle
(d) All the three

123. The carrier of citric acid cycle is:

(a) Malate
(b) Fumarate
(c) Succinate
(d) Oxaloacetate

124. Carbohydrates are polyhydroxy:

(a) Aldehydes
(b) Ketones
(c) Esters
(d) Both (a) and (b)

125. Oxidation of one mole of pyruvate to acetyl CoA leads to the formation of:

(a) 1 mole of ATP
(b) 2 moles of ATP
(c) 3 moles of ATP
(d) 4 moles of ATP

126. One complete kreb cycle starting from oxaloacetate produces how many moles of ATP?

(a) 3
(b) 6
(c) 12
(d) 24

127. Complete oxidation of one free glucose molecule to CO_2 and water under aerobic conditions produce:

(a) 24 moles of ATP
(b) 30 moles of ATP
(c) 38 moles of ATP
(d) 60 moles of ATP

128. The heptose ketose formed in HMP shunt is:

(a) Glucoheptose
(b) Mannoheptose
(c) Galactoheptose
(d) Sedoheptulose

129. Hexose monophosphate pathway of oxidation of glucose is active only in:

(a) Liver
(b) Adipose tissue
(c) Lactating mammary gland
(d) All the three

130. The hydrogen acceptor used in HMP shunt is:

(a) NAD^+ (b) $NADP^+$

(c) Both (a) and (b) (d) Either of the two

131. In one HMP shunt, one molecule of glucose is oxidized with the net generation of:

(a) 35 moles of ATP (b) 36 moles of ATP

(c) 38 moles of ATP (d) 39 moles of ATP

132. During HMP shunt, sedoheptulose-7-phosphate (a C_7 unit) transfers its smaller part to glyceraldehyde-3-phosphate (a C_3 unit) to form:

(a) Ribose-5-phosphate and xylulose-5-phosphate

(b) Ribulose-5-phosphate and xylulose-5-phosphate

(c) Fructose-6-phosphate and erythrose-4-phosphate

(d) Glucose-6-phosphate and erythrose-4-phosphate

133. L-gulonic acid is formed as one of the intermediates in the uronic acid pathway of oxidation of glucose. In man L-gulonic acid is converted into:

(a) Ascorbic acid (b) L-xylulose

(c) Both (a) and (b) (d) Neither of the two

134. In uronic acid pathway, L-xylulose is formed as one of the intermediates. The xylulose of uronic acid pathway may enter HMP shunt as:

(a) L-xylulose (b) D-xylulose

(c) Either (a) or (b) (d) D-ribose

135. In uronic acid pathway, UDPG is oxidized to UPD-glucuronic acid by UDP-dehydrogenase in presence of:

(a) NAD^+ (b) $NADP^+$

(c) FAD^+ (d) $FADP^+$

136. The general formula for polysaccharide:

(a) $(C_6H_{10}O_5)_n$ (b) $(C_6H_{12}O_6)_n$

(c) $(C_6H_{12}O_5)_n$ (d) $(C_6H_{10}O_6)_n$

137. The intermediate in hexose monophosphate shunt:

(a) D-ribulose (b) D-arabinose

(c) D-xylose (d) D-Lyxose

138. Glycosides are found in many:

(a) Vitamins
(b) Drugs
(c) Minerals
(d) Nucleoproteins

139. Erythromycin contains:

(a) Diethyl amino sugars
(b) Triethyl amino sugars
(c) Dimethyl amino sugars
(d) Trimethyl amino sugars

140. The distinguishing test between monosaccharides and disaccharides:

(a) Bial's test
(b) Selivanoff's test
(c) Barfoed's test
(d) Hydrolysis test

141. Glycogen structure includes a branch in between α-glucose units:

(a) 4-10
(b) 6-12
(c) 8-14
(d) 12-18

142. Amylose contains glucose units:

(a) 100-200
(b) 200-300
(c) 300-400
(d) 500-600

143. N-acetyl neuraminic acid is an example of:

(a) Sialic acid
(b) Mucic acid
(c) Glucuronic acid
(d) Hippuric acid

144. The molecular weight of hyaluronic acid in millions ranges from:

(a) 1-2
(b) 1-4
(c) 1-6
(d) 1-8

145. In place of glucuronic acid chondroitin sulphate B contains:

(a) Gluconic acid
(b) Gulonic acid
(c) Iduronic acid
(d) Sulphonic acid

146. Heparin has a molecular weight of about:

(a) 14,000
(b) 15,000
(c) 16,000
(d) 17,000

147. Blood group substances consist of:

(a) Lactose
(b) Maltose
(c) Fucose
(d) Mucose

148. The component of cartilage and cornea is:

(a) Keratan sulphate
(b) Chondroitin sulphate
(c) Cadmium sulphate
(d) None of them

149. Salivary amylase is activated by:

(a) Na^+ (b) K^+

(c) HCO^-_3 (d) Cl^-

150. Benedict's test is less likely to give positive results with concentrated urine due to the action of:

(a) Urea (b) Uric acid

(c) Ammonium sulphates (d) Phosphates

151. Active transport of sugar is depressed by the agent:

(a) Oxaloacetate (b) Fumarate

(c) Malonate (d) Succinate

152. UDPG is essential for the synthesis of:

(a) Lactose (b) Maltose

(c) Sucrose (d) Starch

153. In galactosemic individuals UDP galactose is formed by epimerization from:

(a) Glucose (b) UDP glucose

(c) CDP glucose (d) ITP glucose

154. Galactose is phosphorylated by galactokinase to form:

(a) Galactose-6-phosphate (b) Galactose 1, 6-diphosphate

(c) Galactose-1-phosphate (d) All of them

155. Fructokinase is present in:

(a) Intestine (b) Adipose tissue

(c) Heart (d) Brain

156. Pyruvate is accumulated by the dietary deficiency of:

(a) Vitamin B_6 (b) Folic acid

(c) Vitamin B_{12} (d) Thiamine

157. In liver glyceraldehyde-3-phosphate is converted to:

(a) Glycol (b) Formaldehyde

(c) Formic acid (d) Glycerol

158. Phosphoglycerate kinase responsible for the conversion of 1,3-diphosphoglycerate to 3-phosphoglycerate is inhibited by:

(a) Arsenate (b) Fumarate

(c) Citrate (d) Cyanate

159. The reduced lipoate is re-oxidized by:

(a) NAD^+ (b) $NADP^+$

(c) FAD^+ (d) FMN

160. The approximate number of molecules of pyruvate denhyrogenase in pyruvate dehydrogenase complex:

(a) 19 (b) 29

(c) 39 (d) 49

161. The reactions involving succinyl CoA to succinate requires:

(a) CDP (b) ADP

(c) GDP (d) $NADP^+$

162. The carrier of citric acid cycle:

(a) Succinate (b) Fumarate

(c) Malate (d) Oxaloacetate

163. By killiani-Fischer synthesis, chain length of an aldolase can be increased by:

(a) 1 C-atom (b) 2 C-atom

(c) 3 C-atom (d) None of them

164. Racemic mixture contains D and L isomer in:

(a) Equal concentration (b) Unequal concentration

(c) Both (a) and (b) (d) None of them

165. Sugars forming 5-membered rings are called:

(a) Furanoses (b) Pyranoses

(c) Both (a) and (b) (d) None of them

166. Fructose on reduction produces:

(a) Mannitol (b) Sorbitol

(c) Both (a) and (b) (d) None of them

167. Galactose forms a different osazone owing to carbon number in the structure:

(a) 4 (b) 3

(c) 2 (d) None of them

168. Amylopectin chains have at least:

(a) 80 branches (b) 70 branches

(c) 60 branches (d) None of them

169. Fructose is absorbed at a lower rate than:

(a) Galactose (b) Glucose

(c) Both (a) and (b) (d) None of them

170. In muscles glycogen synthetase exists in 2 forms:

(a) Synthetase D (b) Synthetase 1

(c) Both (a) and (b) (d) None of them

171. Glycogen synthetase is stimulated by:

(a) Insulin (b) Glucose

(c) Both (a) and (b) (d) None of them

172. In liver phosphorylase exists in the form:

(a) Active (b) Inactive

(c) Both (a) and (b) (d) None of them

173. In muscle phosphorylase is present in two forms:

(a) Phosphorylase a (b) Phosphorylase b

(c) Both (a) and (b) (d) None of them

174. A muscle when contracts under unaerobic conditions principal end products are:

(a) Pyruvate (b) Lactate

(c) Both (a) and (b) (d) None of them

175. In the urine of patient suffering from glycosuria, are present:

(a) Ketone bodies (b) Glucose

(c) Both (a) and (b) (d) None of them

176. The key enzymes of glycolysis are:

(a) Glucokinase (b) Pyruvate kinase

(c) Phosphofructokinase (d) All of them

177. cAMP dependent protein kinase is activated by the hormone:

(a) Epinephrine (b) Glucagon

(c) Both (a) and (b) (d) None of them

178. Phosphofructokinase-1 is inhibited by:

(a) ATP (b) Citrate

(c) Both (a) and (b) (d) None of them

179. The main function of TCA cycle is to provide energy through:

(a) Respiratory chain
(b) Oxidative phosphorylation
(c) Both (a) and (b)
(d) None of them

180. Lactate formed by fructolysis is completely oxidized to:

(a) CO_2
(b) H_2O
(c) Both (a) and (b)
(d) None of them

181. The rate limiting step is mainly regulated by the cytoplasmic levels of:

(a) $NADP^+$
(b) NADPH
(c) Both (a) and (b)
(d) None of them

182. The synthesis of pyruvate carboxylase is stimulated by the hormones:

(a) Glucagon
(b) Epinephrine
(c) Gluco-corticoids
(d) All of them

183. The control point in glycogen metabolism involves a cycle of phosphorylation and dephosphorylaton catalyzed by the enzymes:

(a) Phosphorylase
(b) Glycogen synthase
(c) Both (a) and (b)
(d) None of them

184. The key enzymes of the TCA cycle are:

(a) Citrate synthase
(b) Isocitrate dehydrogenase
(c) α-ketoglutarate dehydrogenase
(d) All of them

185. Citrate synthase is allosterically inhibited by:

(a) ATP
(b) Long chain fatty acyl CoA
(c) Both (a) and (b)
(d) None of them

186. The key enzymes of gluconeogenesis are:

(a) Pyruvate carboxylase
(b) Fructose-1,6-diphosphatase
(c) Glucose-6-phosphatase
(d) All of them

187. Fructose-1, 6-diphosphatase is activated by:

(a) ATP
(b) Citrate
(c) Both (a) and (b)
(d) None of them

188. Galactosemia may be responsible for:

(a) Liver enlargement
(b) Opacity in the optic lens
(c) Death
(d) All of them

189. Galactosemia is an inborn error by metabolism, which is characterized by:

(a) Non-accumulation of high concentration of galactose-1- phosphate in RBCs

(b) Accumulation of high concentration of galactose-1- P in RBCs

(c) Accumulation of high concentration of glucose-1- P in RBCs

(d) None of them

190. Gluconeogenesis is a process by which glucose is synthesized from:

(a) Alanine
(b) Pyruvic acid
(c) Lactic acid
(d) All of them

191. Symptoms of dibetes insipidus include:

(a) Increase in fluid intake
(b) Large quantity of urine
(c) Urine of low specific gravity
(d) All of them

192. Ptyalin acts on:

(a) Starch
(b) Glycogen
(c) Both (a) and (b)
(d) All of them

193. Glycogenolysis is a process by which glycogen is synthesized from:

(a) Pyruvic acid
(b) Lactic acid
(c) Glucose
(d) All of them

194. The intestinal mucosal cells secrete a mixture – succus- entericus which contains:

(a) Maltase
(b) Sucrase
(c) Lactase
(d) All of them

195. Glycogenolysis is a process by which glycogen in muscles finally broken down to produce:

(a) Glucose-6-phosphate
(b) Pyruvic acid
(c) Lactic acid
(d) Glucose

196. Main site of gluconeogenesis is:

(a) Brain
(b) Lung
(c) Liver
(d) Pancreas

197. Main sites of glycogenesis are:

(a) Liver
(b) Muscles
(c) Both (a) and (b)
(d) None of them

198. In HMP shunt, ribulose-5-phosphate is isomerized to a mixture of ketopentoses, which are:

(a) Ribose-5-P
(b) Xylulose-5-phosphate
(c) Both (a) and (b)
(d) None of them

199. A c-atom is said to be asymmetric when it is attached to atoms/groups in number:

(a) 2
(b) 3
(c) 4
(d) None of them

200. In TCA cycle when succinyl CoA gets converted to succinic acid; at the stage an energy rich compound formed is:

(a) Guanosine triphosphate
(b) Adenosine monophosphate
(c) Adenosine diphosphate
(d) None of them

Answer Key

1	(c)	26	(d)	51	(c)	76	(a)
2	(d)	27	(c)	52	(b)	77	(a)
3	(c)	28	(d)	53	(b)	78	(c)
4	(b)	29	(d)	54	(b)	79	(a)
5	(d)	30	(c)	55	(d)	80	(c)
6	(b)	31	(b)	56	(a)	81	(c)
7	(a)	32	(c)	57	(a)	82	(a)
8	(a)	33	(c)	58	(a)	83	(c)
9	(a)	34	(c)	59	(a)	84	(a)
10	(a)	35	(b)	60	(c)	85	(d)
11	(a)	36	(c)	61	(b)	86	(a)
12	(b)	37	(c)	62	(c)	87	(b)
13	(a)	38	(a)	63	(a)	88	(c)
14	(a)	39	(d)	64	(c)	89	(b)
15	(a)	40	(a)	65	(c)	90	(b)
16	(b)	41	(b)	66	(c)	91	(b)
17	(b)	42	(c)	67	(a)	92	(d)
18	(c)	43	(d)	68	(c)	93	(a)
19	(c)	44	(a)	69	(d)	94	(b)
20	(a)	45	(c)	70	(d)	95	(d)
21	(b)	46	(c)	71	(a)	96	(c)
22	(b)	47	(c)	72	(a)	97	(b)
23	(d)	48	(c)	73	(a)	98	(a)
24	(d)	49	(a)	74	(c)	99	(c)
25	(b)	50	(c)	75	(a)	100	(d)

101	(c)	126	(c)	151	(c)	176	(d)
102	(a)	127	(c)	152	(a)	177	(c)
103	(c)	128	(d)	153	(b)	178	(c)
104	(b)	129	(d)	154	(c)	179	(c)
105	(a)	130	(b)	155	(a)	180	(c)
106	(c)	131	(a)	156	(d)	181	(c)
107	(b)	132	(c)	157	(d)	182	(d)
108	(a)	133	(b)	158	(a)	183	(c)
109	(c)	134	(b)	159	(c)	184	(d)
110	(c)	135	(a)	160	(b)	185	(c)
111	(d)	136	(a)	161	(c)	186	(d)
112	(c)	137	(a)	162	(d)	187	(c)
113	(b)	138	(b)	163	(a)	188	(d)
114	(d)	139	(a)	164	(b)	189	(b)
115	(c)	140	(c)	165	(a)	190	(d)
116	(a)	141	(d)	166	(c)	191	(d)
117	(d)	142	(c)	167	(a)	192	(c)
118	(d)	143	(a)	168	(a)	193	(c)
119	(c)	144	(b)	169	(c)	194	(d)
120	(d)	145	(c)	170	(c)	195	(a)
121	(a)	146	(d)	171	(c)	196	(c)
122	(d)	147	(c)	172	(c)	197	(c)
123	(d)	148	(a)	173	(c)	198	(c)
124	(c)	149	(d)	174	(c)	199	(c)
125	(c)	150	(b)	175	(b)	200	(a)

Chapter 3

Lipids and their Metabolism

1. **Lipids are soluble in:**
   (a) Water (b) Organic solvents
   (c) Both (a) and (b) (d) None of them
2. **Esters of long chain fatty acids with long chain monohydric alcohol are known as:**
   (a) Fats (b) Waxes
   (c) Both (a) and (b) (d) None of them
3. **Naturally occurring fatty acids usually contain:**
   (a) Even number of carbon-atom (b) Odd number of carbon-atom
   (c) Both (a) and (b) (d) None of them
4. **Animal fats mainly contain:**
   (a) Stearic and palmitic acid (b) Linoleic and linolenic acid
   (c) Both (a) and (b) (d) None of them
5. **Essential fatty acids contain:**
   (a) Two double bonds (b) Three double bonds
   (c) Four double bonds (d) All the three
6. **Essential fatty acids are found mainly in:**
   (a) Corn oil (b) Cotton seed oil
   (c) Sunflower oil (d) All the three

7. Δ^8 indicates a double bond between carbon-atoms:

(a) 7 and 8
(b) 8 and 9
(c) 8 and 10
(d) 6 and 8

8. Arachidonic acid contains the number of double bonds:

(a) 2
(b) 3
(c) 4
(d) 5

9. Prostaglandins are synthesized from:

(a) Arachidonic acid
(b) Oleic acid
(c) Linoleic acid
(d) Linolenic acid

10. Chaulmoogric acid was used in early days in the treatment of:

(a) Oedema
(b) Nephritis
(c) Leprosy
(d) All of them

11. Essential fatty acids retard:

(a) Atherosclerosis
(b) Diabetes mellitus
(c) Nephritis
(d) Oedema

12. Hydrolysis of fat by alkali is called:

(a) Saponification number
(b) Saponification
(c) Both (a) and (b)
(d) None of them

13. Rancidity is more pronounced in animal fats than in plant fats because:

(a) Animal fats contain higher amount of acids
(b) Animal fats have higher percentage of saturated fatty acids
(c) Plant fats contain certain antioxidant which prevent oxidation
(d) None of the above

14. Lecithins combine with protein to form:

(a) Phosphoprotein
(b) Glycoprotein
(c) Lipoprotein
(d) Mucoprotein

15. Protein molecule of lipoprotein is:

(a) Preprotein
(b) Postprotein
(c) Apoprotein
(d) Pseudoprotein

16. Apoprotein constitutes chylomicrons in per cent:

(a) 0.4
(b) 0.6
(c) 0.8
(d) 1.0

17. Gangliosides are glycolipids occurring in:

(a) Liver (b) Brain

(c) Kidney (d) Muscle

18. In gangliosides, sugar protein may be:

(a) Acetylated amino sugars (b) Sialic acid

(c) Both (a) and (b) (d) None of them

19. Lipoprotein present in cell membrane is:

(a) Hydrophilic (b) Hydrophobic

(c) Both (a) and (b) (d) None of them

20. The density of Lipoprotein increases as the protein content:

(a) Increases (b) Decreases

(c) Remains same (d) None of them

21. Lecithin contains a nitrogenous base called as:

(a) Ethanolamine (b) Choline

(c) Inositol (d) All of them

22. Cephalins are compound lipids which contain:

(a) Ethanolamine (b) Myoinositol

(c) Both (a) and (b) (d) None of them

23. In sphingomyelins, the alcohol moiety is:

(a) Glycerol (b) Glycol

(c) Sphingosine (d) All of them

24. Name the test employed to check the purity of butter through the estimation of volatile fatty acids:

(a) Iodine number (b) Reichert-Meissel number

(c) Saponification number (d) Acid number

25. The lipoprotein possessing the highest quality of phospholipid:

(a) HDL (b) LDL

(c) VLDL (d) Chylomicrons

26. Esterification of cholesterol occurs at carbon position:

(a) 1 (b) 2

(c) 3 (d) 4

27. One of the following is an amphipathic lipid:

(a) Phospholipid (b) Fatty acid
(c) Bile salts (d) All of them

28. The following substance is ketogenic:

(a) Fatty acid (b) Leucine
(c) Lysine (d) All of them

29. Hypercholestermia is observed in the disorder:

(a) Hypothyroidism (b) Diabetes mellitus
(c) Nephrotic syndrome (d) All of them

30. The main source of cholesterol is:

(a) Animal fats (b) Vegetable fats
(c) Egg Yolk (d) All of them

31. Soap is:

(a) A mixture of salts of fatty acids (b) A salt of glycerol
(c) A mixture of ethers (d) All of them

32. Rancidity of butter is prevented by the addition of:

(a) Tocopherols (b) Vitamin D
(c) Biotin (d) Copper

33. The smell of fat turns rancid due to the presence of:

(a) Vitamin E (b) Quinone
(c) Cholesterol (d) Volatile fatty acids

34. All of the following are constituents of gaglioside molecule except:

(a) Glycerol (b) Sialic acid
(c) Sphingosine (d) Hexose sugar

35. The number of mg of KOH required to neutralize free fatty acids present in 1g fat or oil is known as:

(a) RM number (b) Acid number
(c) Iodine number (d) Saponification number

36. Which one is steroid hormone?

(a) Androgens (b) Estrogens
(c) Corticoids (d) All of them

37. Fat is stored in:

(a) Liver (b) Kidney
(c) Adipose tissue (d) All the three

38. Digestion of fat starts in:

(a) Mouth (b) Stomach
(c) Small intestine (d) Large intestine

39. Lipids are emulsified by the action of:

(a) Lipoproteins (b) Cholesterol
(c) Ergosterol (d) Bile salts

40. Lipase present in stomach can not hydrolyse fats due to:

(a) Alkalinity (b) Acidity
(c) High acidity (d) Neutrality

41. Majority of absorbed fats appear in the form of:

(a) HDL (b) LDL
(c) VLDL (d) Chylomicrons

42. Fatty acids are oxidized mainly by:

(a) α-oxidation (b) β-oxidation
(c) γ-oxidation (d) All of them

43. During oxidation, long chain fatty acids are first converted to acyl-coenzyme A in the:

(a) Cytosol (b) Mitochondria
(c) Lysosomes (d) Microsomes

44. Activation of lower fatty acids occurs within the:

(a) Cytosol (b) Mitochondria
(c) Lysosomes (d) Microsomes

45. The enzyme thiokinase catalyzing the activation of the fatty acids require:

(a) Ca^{++} (b) Mg^{++}
(c) Mn^{++} (d) K^{+}

46. Acyl-CoA is converted to α, β unsaturated acyl CoA by the enzyme acyl-CoA dehydrogenase in presence of co-enzyme:

(a) NAD^{+} (b) $NADP^{+}$
(c) FAD^{+} (d) ATP

47. During one set of β-oxidation of a fatty acid, number of carbon atoms removed is:

(a) 1
(b) 2
(c) 3
(d) Not definite

48. The final product of β-oxidation of an odd-numbered carboxylic acid is:

(a) Acetyl CoA
(b) Propionyl CoA
(c) Either of the two
(d) None of them

49. Number of ATP molecules liberated during the oxidation of one mole of palmitic acid to CO_2 and H_2O is:

(a) 128
(b) 129
(c) 130
(d) 131

50. Under normal conditions the fate of acetyl-CoA formed by the oxidation of fatty acyl CoA:

(a) Conversion to acetone
(b) Conversion to acetoacetate
(c) Entry to citric acid cycle
(d) None of them

51. Normal concentration of ketone bodies in mg percent in blood does not exceed:

(a) 1
(b) 1.5
(c) 2.0
(d) 2.5

52. When the concentration of ketone bodies in blood increases, condition is known as:

(a) Ketonuria
(b) Ketonemia
(c) Ketosis
(d) Ketogenesis

53. Ketosis generally occurs in:

(a) Nephritis
(b) Oedema
(c) Infective hepatic disease
(d) None of them

54. Enzymes responsible for ketone body formation are found mainly in:

(a) Mitochondria
(b) Extrahepatic tissue
(c) Nucleus
(d) Chromosomes

55. Under prolonged starvation brain takes energy from:

(a) Carbohydrates
(b) Fats
(c) Acetoacetate
(d) Proteins

56. Fatty acid oxidation takes place in:

(a) Cytosol
(b) Mitochondria
(c) Microsomes
(d) All of them

57. Fatty acid synthesis occurs in:

(a) Cytosol
(b) Mitochondria
(c) Microsomes
(d) All of them

58. Lengthening of carbon chain of fatty acid takes place in:

(a) Cytosol
(b) Mitochondria
(c) Mitochondria and microsomes
(d) Microsomes

59. Lengthening of fatty acid in mitochondria and microsomes takes place by the addition of:

(a) Acetyl CoA
(b) Propionyl CoA
(c) Acetyl CoA and propionyl CoA, respectively
(d) None of them

60. Acetyl CoA formed in the mitochondria migrates to cytosol in the form of:

(a) Acetyl CoA itself
(b) Oxaloacetate
(c) Citrate
(d) Malate

61. How many moles of NADPH are generated for the migration of 1 mole of NADPH from mitochondria to cytosol?

(a) 1
(b) 2
(c) 3
(d) 4

62. Acetyl CoA carboxylase involved in the carboxylation of acetyl CoA contains:

(a) Biotin
(b) Cyanocobalamin
(c) Pyridoxal
(d) None of them

63. The reductive steps in the fatty acid synthesis takes place in presence of the coenzyme:

(a) NAD^+
(b) Reduced NAD
(c) $NADP^+$
(d) Reduced NADP

64. The dehydrogenating steps in the β-oxidation of fatty acids utilize:

(a) NAD^+
(b) $NADP^+$
(c) NADH
(d) NADPH

65. The intermediates in fatty acid synthesis are covalently linked to:

(a) Acyl carrier protein (b) Coenzyme A
(c) Coenzyme Q (d) None of them

66. Phospholipids help in the oxidation of:

(a) Glycerol (b) Fatty acids
(c) Glycerophosphate (d) None of the above

67. The introduction of double bond and chain elongation system of polyunsaturated fatty acids are greatly diminished in absence of:

(a) Glucagon (b) Insulin
(c) Epinephrine (d) Thyroxine

68. The prostaglandins are derived from a common structure based on prostanoic acid containing:

(a) 16 carbon-atoms (b) 18 carbon-atoms
(c) 20 carbon-atoms (d) 22 carbon-atoms

69. The carbon chain of prostanoic acid has a cyclic ring in the middle. It is:

(a) 4-membered ring (b) 5-membered ring
(c) 6-membered ring (d) 7-membered ring

70. All active prostaglandins have a common double bond which lies:

(a) Between C_{17} and C_{18} and has cis-configuration
b) Between C_{17} and C_{18} and has trans configuration
(c) Between C_{13} and C_{14} and has cis-configuration
(d) Between C_{13} and C_{14} and has trans configuration

71. Prostaglandins are liberated in the circulation by stimulation of:

(a) Anterior pituitary gland (b) Posterior pituitary gland
(c) Adrenal body (d) Thyroid gland

72. Synthesis of prostaglandins is inhibited by:

(a) Aspirin (b) Fluoride ion
(c) Cyanide ion (d) Arsenite ion

73. Prostaglandins are used for:

(a) Induction of menstruation (b) Prevention of conception
(c) Termination of pregnancy (d) All the three cases

74. Prostaglandins increase intestinal motility and cause:

(a) Loose motion
(b) Diarrhoea
(c) Dysentry
(d) Constipation

75. The normal concentration of cholesterol in plasma is:

(a) 100mg/100ml
(b) 150mg/100ml
(c) 250mg/100ml
(d) 300mg/100ml

76. The blood cholesterol level is increased in the deficiency of:

(a) Vitamin B_2
(b) Vitamin B_6
(c) Vitamin D
(d) Inositol

77. Ingested cholesterol is absorbed from the intestine and incorporated into:

(a) Chylomicrons
(b) VLDL
(c) Both (a) and (b)
(d) HDL

78. Cholesterol contains 27 carbon-atoms which are derived from:

(a) CO_2 and glucose molecule
(b) Higher fatty acid molecules
(c) Acetate molecules
(d) Coenzyme A molecule

79. Of the 27 carbon-atoms of cholesterol, how many are derived from the CH_3-group of the acetate molecule?

(a) All the 27
(b) 13
(c) 14
(d) 15

80. The most important site for cholesterol synthesis is:

(a) Intestine
(b) Liver
(c) Kidney
(d) Blood

81. Biosynthesis of cholesterol in liver is suppressed by:

(a) Dietary cholesterol
(b) Fasting
(c) Both (a) and (b)
(d) None of them

82. Fatty liver is caused by:

(a) CH_3Cl
(b) CCl_4
(c) $MgSO_4$
(d) CH_3COOH

83. Fatty appearance and enlargement of the liver are caused by:

(a) Pregnancy
(b) Nephritis
(c) Abortion
(d) Toxaemia of pregnancy

84. Fatty liver results in the deficiency of:

(a) Stearic acid
(b) Caproic acid
(c) Vitamin A
(d) Pantothenic acid

85. Triacylglycerol is accumulated even in normal rate of fatty acid synthesis by the deficiency of:

(a) Calcium
(b) Vitamin A
(c) Vitamin C
(d) Lipotropic factor

86. Only physiologically significant site for the formation of ketone bodies is:

(a) Liver
(b) Muscles
(c) Kidney
(d) Intestine

87. In the blood severe atherosclerosis is accompanied by the prolonged elevated levels of:

(a) LDL
(b) VLDL
(c) Both (a) and (b)
(d) None of them

88. The principal organ for synthesis of cholesterol is:

(a) Liver
(b) Kidney
(c) Intestine
(d) Muscle

89. LDL is formed from:

(a) VLDL
(b) Chylomicrons
(c) Both (a) and (b)
(d) None of them

90. HDL is synthesized and secreted from:

(a) Liver
(b) Intestine
(c) Both (a) and (b)
(d) None of them

91. In HDL predominant lipids are:

(a) Phospholipids
(b) Sphingolipids
(c) Both (a) and (b)
(d) None of them

92. Phospholipids act as carrier of:

(a) Inorganic ions
(b) Organic ions
(c) Both (a) and (b)
(d) None of them

93. The energy metabolism of ruminants is focused on the utilization of:

(a) Volatile fatty acids
(b) Non-volatile fatty acids
(c) Chylomicrons
(d) LDLP

94. CPT participates in the biosynthesis of:

(a) Gangliosides
(b) Sphingomyelin
(c) Phosphoglycerides
(d) All of them

95. Respiratory distress syndrome in infants is characterized by:

(a) Presence of dipalmitoyl lecithin
(b) Absence of dipalmitoyl lecithin
(c) Both (a) and (b)
(d) None of them

96. Effector hormone for lipogenesis is:

(a) Insulin
(b) Glucocorticoid
(c) Thyroxine
(d) Vasopressin

97. Bile is secreted by:

(a) Liver
(b) Stomach
(c) Pancreas
(d) Intestine

98. Myristic acid is:

(a) Fatty acylated protein
(b) Fatty acid
(c) Both (a) and (b)
(d) None of them

99. Ketonemia in diabetes is due to:

(a) Increased lipolysis
(b) Accelerated hepatic gluconeogenesis
(c) Both (a) and (b)
(d) None of them

100. In spontaneous ketosis, milk production is:

(a) Decreased
(b) Increased
(c) Remains same
(d) All of them

101. Source of essential fatty acids is:

(a) Butter
(b) Mustard oil
(c) Desi ghee
(d) Safflower oil

102. Fatty acid synthesis requires:

(a) NAD^+
(b) FAD
(c) NADPH
(d) TPP

103. In cholesterol biosynthesis, acetoacetyl Coenzyme A is converted to:

(a) HMG CoA (b) Mevalonic acid

(c) Acetyl CoA (d) Squalene

104. Oxidation of choline leads to the formation of:

(a) Betaine (b) Ethanolamine

(c) Cysteine (d) Cystine

105. Phenylketonuria is characterized by:

(a) Gastritis (b) Pain in joints

(c) Nephrons (d) Mental retardation

106. Due to mobilities of lipids, lipid bilayer can be considered to be a:

(a) One dimensional fluid (b) Two dimensional fluid

(c) Both (a) and (b) (d) None of them

107. Amphipathic possess in its structure:

(a) Hydrophobic groups (b) Hydrophilic groups

(c) Both (a) and (b) (d) None of them

108. HDL is correlated with coronary heart disease:

(a) Inversely (b) Directly

(c) Both (a) and (b) (d) None of them

109. Fats are solid at:

(a) 10°C (b) 20°C

(c) 30°C (d) 40°C

110. The combination of an amino alcohol, fatty acid and sialic acid form:

(a) Phospholipids (b) Sulpholipids

(c) Glycolipids (d) Amino lipids

111. Development of rancidity is prevented by:

(a) Vitamin A (b) Vitamin E

(c) Vitamin C (d) None of them

112. The number of millilitre of 0.1N KOH required to neutralize the insoluble fatty acids from 5 grams of fat is called:

(a) Acid number (b) Acetyl number

(c) Halogenation (d) Polenske number

113. The rate of fatty acid oxidation is increased by:

(a) Phospholipids (b) Glycolipids

(c) Amino lipids (d) All of them

114. Cardiolipin found in mitochondria is formed from:

(a) Lipositol (b) Phosphatidyl ethanolamine

(c) Phosphatidyl glycerol (d) None of them

115. Lecithin contains unsaturated fatty acid at position:

(a) α - (b) α and β

(c) β - (d) None of them

116. Lecithins are soluble in ordinary fat solvents except:

(a) Benzene (b) Ethyl alcohol

(c) Methyl alcohol (d) Acetone

117. When lecithins exposed to air become:

(a) Black (b) Brown

(c) Red (d) Yellow

118. Instead of ester link plasmalogens possess an ether link in position:

(a) α- (b) β -

(c) γ - (d) None of them

119. The alkyl radical in plasmalogen is an alcohol:

(a) Saturated (b) Unsaturated

(c) Both (a) and (b) (d) None of them

120. The concentrations of sphingomyelins are increased by:

(a) Gaucher's disease (b) Fabry's disease

(c) Febrile disease (d) Niemann-Pick disease

121. Glycolipids contain an amino alcohol:

(a) Sphingosine (b) Isosphingosine

(c) Both (a) and (b) (d) None of them

122. Cerebrosides may also be classified as:

(a) Sphingolipids (b) Sulpholipids

(c) Amino lipids (d) Glycolipids

123. Most of the gangliosides contain sialic acid upto the molecular number:

(a) 1 (b) 2

(c) 3 (d) 4

124. The percentage of triacylglycerol of lipoproteins:

(a) 30 (b) 35

(c) 40 (d) 45

125. Cholesterol and cholesteryl esters in per cent present in lipoproteins:

(a) 15 (b) 20

(c) 25 (d) 28

126. Lipoproteins may be identified more accurately by means of:

(a) Electrophoresis (b) Centrifugation

(c) Immuno electrophoresis (d) Ultracentrifugation

127. Very low density lipoproteins are also known as:

(a) β-Lipoproteins (b) Pre-β-lipoproteins

(c) α-Lipoproteins (d) None of them

128. The β-lipoprotein fraction increases in severe:

(a) Diabetes mellitus (b) Uremia

(c) Nephritis (d) Muscular dystrophy

129. Sulpholipids have been isolated from:

(a) Heart (b) Liver

(c) Brain (d) Intestine

130. The number of carbon atoms in decanoic acid present in butter:

(a) 6 (b) 8

(c) 10 (d) 12

131. Lignoceric acid present in peanut oil contains carbon atoms:

(a) 18 (b) 20

(c) 22 (d) 24

132. The iodine number of essential fatty acids of vegetable oils:

(a) High (b) Very high

(c) Very low (d) Low

133. The shape of arachidonic acid:

(a) L (b) M

(c) U (d) V

134. The example of cardiac glycosides:

(a) Digitonin (b) Strobanthin

(c) Lycopyll (d) Digitalis

135. The reduction product of cholesterol by bacteria in the intestine occurs in feces:

(a) Ergosterol (b) Demosterol

(c) Coprosterol (d) Lanosterol

136. Lieberman-Burchard reaction is performed to detect:

(a) Cholesterol (b) Glycerol

(c) Fatty acid (d) Vitamin D

137. The free glycerol of the total amount of triacylglycerol in the intestinal lumen is present in per cent about:

(a) 16 (b) 18

(c) 20 (d) 22

138. More metabolic water is available on oxidation of:

(a) Fatty acids (b) Glycerol

(c) Both (a) and (b) (d) None of them

139. Long chain acyl-CoA penetrates mitochondria in presence of:

(a) Palmitate (b) Carnitine

(c) Sorbitol (d) DNP

140. ω-oxidation takes place by the hydroxylase in microsomes involving:

(a) Cytochrome b (b) Cytochrome C

(c) Cytochrome P-450 (d) Cytochrome a_3

141. Carboxylation of acetyl-CoA to malonyl-CoA takes place in presence of:

(a) FAD^+ (b) Biotin

(c) NAD^+ (d) $NADP^+$

142. Malonyl-CoA reacts with the central:

(a) –SH group (b) $-NH_2$ group

(c) –COOH group (d) $-CH_2OH$ group

143. In adipose tissues prostaglandins decrease:

(a) Lipogenesis (b) Ketogenesis

(c) Lipolysis (d) Ketolysis

144. Phospholipase A_1 attacks the ester bond of phospholipids in position:

(a) 1 (b) 2

(c) 3 (d) All of them

145. Phospholipase C releases 1,2-diacylglycerol and a phosphoryl base attacking the ester bond in position:

(a) 1 (b) 2

(c) 3 (d) 4

146. The synthesis of prostaglandins requires the consumption of two molecules of oxygen and two molecules of reduced:

(a) NAD (b) NADP

(c) Glutathione (d) Lipoate

147. Prostaglandins lower cyclic AMP in:

(a) Thyroid (b) Adipose tissues

(c) Platelets (d) Lungs

148. The inhibitory activity of prostaglandins in liver is effective on:

(a) Glycogen synthetase (b) Hexokinase

(c) Phosphorylase (d) Glucose-6-phosphatase

149. The enzyme responsible for the metabolism of prostaglandin is blocked by the introduction of a methyl group at:

(a) C_9 position (b) C_{11} position

(c) C_{13} position (d) C_{15} Position

150. In adipose tissues less glycerol-3-phosphate is formed in:

(a) Diabetes mellitus (b) Nephritis

(c) Coronary thrombosis (d) Heart failure

151. LDL contains the apoprotein:

(a) C-I (b) C-II

(c) C-III (d) B

152. The normal concentration of β-lipoproteins in mg per cent in plasma:

(a) 100 (b) 200

(c) 300 (d) 400

153. The concentration of triacylglycerol in Pre-β-lipoproteins in per cent:

(a) 40 (b) 45

(c) 50 (d) 55

154. Chylomicrons and VLDL both are released from the intestine or hepatic cell by reverse:

(a) Pinocytosis (b) Diffusion

(c) Osmosis (d) Passive diffusion

155. Serum LDL has been found to be increased in:

(a) Obstructive jaundice (b) Hepatic jaundice

(c) Hemolytic jaundice (d) Septicemia

156. The enzyme system for lengthening and shortening for saturing and desaturing fatty acids occurs in:

(a) Intestine (b) Muscle

(c) Kidney (d) Liver

157. The lowered glucokinase leading to diminished fatty acid synthesis in the liver is caused by the effect of:

(a) Feeding (b) Overfeeding

(c) Starvation (d) Diarrhoea

158. The increased levels of plasma free fatty acids resulting from mobilization of fat from:

(a) Muscle (b) Adipose tissue

(c) Kidney (d) Intestine

159. The lipotropic activity is possessed by:

(a) Casein (b) Cellulose

(c) Phospholipids (d) Glycolipids

160. Ketone bodies are utilized in:

(a) Mitochondria (b) Extra hepatic tissue

(c) Nuclei (d) Chromosomes

161. The excretion of ketone bodies in the urine involves the deficiency of:

(a) Na^{+} (b) Fe^{++}

(c) Ca^{++} (d) Mg^{++}

162. Eicosanoids are formed from:

(a) Arachidonate (b) Palmitate

(c) Stearate (d) Butyrate

163. Eicosanoids are derived from:

(a) Linoleic acid (b) Linolenic acid

(c) Arachidonic acid (d) All of them

164. The concentration of smooth muscle is caused by prostaglandins with the minimum concentration of:

(a) 1mg/ml (b) 10mg/ml

(c) 100mg/ml (d) 1ng/ml

165. Leukotrienes are important in:

(a) Allergic reaction
(b) Oxidation reaction
(c) Reduction reaction
(d) Inhibitory reaction

166. The Eskimos have low plasma concentrations of:

(a) Cholesterol
(b) Triacylglycerol
(c) LDL
(d) All of them

167. Prostaglandins increase cAMP in:

(a) Platelets
(b) Thyroid
(c) Corpus luteum
(d) All of them

168. PG_3 and TX_3 inhibit the release of:

(a) Oleic acid
(b) Palmitoleic acid
(c) Palmitic acid
(d) Arachidonic acid

169. Leukotriene C_4 is formed by the addition of:

(a) Ascorbic acid
(b) Glutathione
(c) Glutamate
(d) Aspartate

170. Leukotriene A_4 is metabolized to leukotriene:

(a) C_2
(b) C_3
(c) C_4
(d) D_4

171. Leukotrienes are formed by only:

(a) 5-Lipooxygenase
(b) Lipase
(c) Phospholipase
(d) None of them

172. Leukotrienes are formed in:

(a) Leukocytes
(b) Mastocytoma
(c) Platelets
(d) All of them

173. PGH (Endoperoxide) is converted to prostaglandin:

(a) D
(b) E
(c) F
(d) All of them

174. Cyclooxygenase is termed as:

(a) Inhibiting enzyme
(b) Suicide enzyme
(c) Oxidizing enzyme
(d) Reducing enzyme

175. Lecithins can exist in:

(a) α-form
(b) β-form
(c) Either of the two
(d) Neither of the two

176. Amino lipids are:

(a) Phosphatidyl ethanolamine
(b) Serine
(c) Both (a) and (b)
(d) None of them

177. In the structure of linoleic acid, the unsaturated carbon atoms are at:

(a) Δ^9
(b) Δ^{12}
(c) Both (a) and (b)
(d) None of them

178. The essential fatty acids of vegetable oils have low:

(a) Melting point
(b) Iodine number
(c) Both (a) and (b)
(d) None of them

179. Increased fecal excretion of cholesterol and bile acids is caused by the drug:

(a) Choloxin
(b) Neomycin
(c) Both (a) and (b)
(d) None of them

180. Vitamins able to produce lipotropic effect are:

(a) B_{12}
(b) Folic acid
(c) Both (a) and (b)
(d) None of them

181. Fatty liver causes the metabolic block in the synthesis of lipoproteins from:

(a) Lipid
(b) Apoprotein
(c) Both (a) and (b)
(d) None of them

182. Cyclooxygenase is inhibited by:

(a) Aspirin
(b) Indomethacin
(c) Both (a) and (b)
(d) None of them

183. Tay Sach's disease is characterized by increased accumulation of GM_2 gangliosides in:

(a) Brain
(b) Spleen
(c) Both (a) and (b)
(d) None of them

184. In the form of cholesterol-sterol- carrier protein cholesterol is converted to:

(a) Steroid hormones
(b) Bile acids
(c) Both (a) and (b)
(d) None of them

185. In 'Tangier disease', HDL is:

(a) Absent from plasma (b) Present in plasma

(c) Sometimes present in plasma (d) None of them

186. In the absence of insulin, fat synthesis takes place:

(a) More (b) As usual

(c) Very little (d) None of them

187. When ketosis is evident, fat synthesis gets:

(a) Increased (b) Suppressed

(c) As usual (d) None of them

188. Most important site of fat metabolism is:

(a) Adipose tissue (b) Liver

(c) Intestine (d) All of them

189. Effect of insulin on the rate of fatty acid synthesis *de novo* is:

(a) Rate increased (b) Rate decreased

(c) No effect (d) None of them

190. When carbohydrate is ingested, fat oxidation is:

(a) Reduced (b) No effect

(c) Increased (d) None of them

191. Hydroxymethyl glutaryl CoA synthetase is inhibited by:

(a) Cholesterol (b) α-ketoacids

(c) Methionine (d) Glutamine

192. In severe ketosis, reduction in plasma bicarbonate and the loss of cations in urine is:

(a) Dangerous (b) No effect

(c) Not dangerous (d) None of them

193. The cholesterol which is present in plasma originated largely from:

(a) Hepatic synthesis (b) Renal synthesis

(c) Brain synthesis (d) None of them

194. The fatty acid which predominate in cholesterol are:

(a) Oleic acid (b) Linoleic acid

(c) Both (a) and (b) (d) None of them

195. Arachidonic acid is a precursor of:

(a) Vitamin A
(b) Prostaglandins
(c) Vitamin K
(d) Sex hormones

196. In cholesterol biosynthesis farnesyl pyrophosphate is converted to:

(a) Isopentyl pyrophosphate
(b) Geranyl pyrophosphate
(c) Squalene
(d) None of them

197. In severe ketosis rate of TCA cycle will be:

(a) Decreased
(b) Increased
(c) Remains same
(d) None of them

198. In their structures prostaglandins possess:

(a) Cyclopentane ring
(b) Benzene ring
(c) Cyclopentanoperhydrophenanthrene
(d) None of them

199. In cholesterol biosynthesis, acetoacetyl CoA is converted to:

(a) Acetyl CoA
(b) Mevalonic acid
(c) β-hydroxy β-methyl glutaryl CoA
(d) Squalene

200. In the biosyntehsis of cholic acid, cholesterol gets firstly converted to:

(a) 7-hydroxycholesterol
(b) Chenodeoxycholic acid
(c) 7-dehydrocholesterol
(d) None of them

Answer Key

1	(b)	26	(c)	51	(a)	76	(b)
2	(b)	27	(d)	52	(b)	77	(c)
3	(a)	28	(b)	53	(c)	78	(c)
4	(a)	29	(a)	54	(a)	79	(d)
5	(d)	30	(a)	55	(c)	80	(b)
6	(d)	31	(a)	56	(b)	81	(c)
7	(b)	32	(a)	57	(a)	82	(b)
8	(c)	33	(d)	58	(c)	83	(d)
9	(a)	34	(a)	59	(c)	84	(d)
10	(c)	35	(b)	60	(b)	85	(d)
11	(a)	36	(d)	61	(a)	86	(a)
12	(b)	37	(c)	62	(a)	87	(c)
13	(c)	38	(c)	63	(d)	88	(a)
14	(c)	39	(d)	64	(a)	89	(c)
15	(c)	40	(c)	65	(a)	90	(c)
16	(d)	41	(d)	66	(b)	91	(a)
17	(b)	42	(b)	67	(b)	92	(a)
18	(b)	43	(a)	68	(c)	93	(a)
19	(a)	44	(b)	69	(b)	94	(d)
20	(b)	45	(b)	70	(d)	95	(a)
21	(b)	46	(c)	71	(c)	96	(a)
22	(a)	47	(b)	72	(c)	97	(a)
23	(c)	48	(b)	73	(d)	98	(a)
24	(b)	49	(b)	74	(a)	99	(d)
25	(a)	50	(c)	75	(a)	100	(a)

101	**(d)**	**126**	**(c)**	**151**	**(d)**	**176**	**(c)**
102	**(c)**	**127**	**(b)**	**152**	**(c)**	**177**	**(c)**
103	**(b)**	**128**	**(a)**	**153**	**(c)**	**178**	**(c)**
104	**(b)**	**129**	**(c)**	**154**	**(a)**	**179**	**(c)**
105	**(d)**	**130**	**(c)**	**155**	**(a)**	**180**	**(c)**
106	**(b)**	**131**	**(d)**	**156**	**(d)**	**181**	**(c)**
107	**(b)**	**132**	**(d)**	**157**	**(c)**	**182**	**(c)**
108	**(a)**	**133**	**(c)**	**158**	**(b)**	**183**	**(c)**
109	**(b)**	**134**	**(b)**	**159**	**(a)**	**184**	**(c)**
110	**(c)**	**135**	**(c)**	**160**	**(b)**	**185**	**(a)**
111	**(b)**	**136**	**(a)**	**161**	**(a)**	**186**	**(c)**
112	**(d)**	**137**	**(d)**	**162**	**(a)**	**187**	**(b)**
113	**(a)**	**138**	**(a)**	**163**	**(d)**	**188**	**(d)**
114	**(c)**	**139**	**(b)**	**164**	**(d)**	**189**	**(a)**
115	**(c)**	**140**	**(c)**	**165**	**(a)**	**190**	**(a)**
116	**(d)**	**141**	**(b)**	**166**	**(d)**	**191**	**(a)**
117	**(b)**	**142**	**(a)**	**167**	**(d)**	**192**	**(a)**
118	**(a)**	**143**	**(a)**	**168**	**(d)**	**193**	**(a)**
119	**(b)**	**144**	**(a)**	**169**	**(b)**	**194**	**(c)**
120	**(d)**	**145**	**(c)**	**170**	**(c)**	**195**	**(b)**
121	**(c)**	**146**	**(c)**	**171**	**(a)**	**196**	**(c)**
122	**(a)**	**147**	**(b)**	**172**	**(d)**	**197**	**(a)**
123	**(c)**	**148**	**(a)**	**173**	**(d)**	**198**	**(a)**
124	**(d)**	**149**	**(d)**	**174**	**(b)**	**199**	**(c)**
125	**(a)**	**150**	**(a)**	**175**	**(c)**	**200**	**(a)**

Chapter 4

Amino Acids, Proteins and their Metabolism

1. **Amino acids capable of being utilized by human body belongs to:**
   (a) D-series (b) L-series
   (c) Both (a) and (b) (d) None of them
2. **All α-amino acids are optically active except:**
   (a) Glycine (b) Alanine
   (c) Serine (d) Phenylalanine
3. **Amino acids have net zero charge at:**
   (a) Isoelectric point (b) Every pH
   (c) Both (a) and (b) (d) None of them
4. **Which of the following is not essential amino acid?**
   (a) Leucine (b) Valine
   (c) Threonine (d) Alanine
5. **Amino acids exist as:**
   (a) Cations (b) Anions
   (c) Zwitter ions (d) None of them

6. **The number of amino acids present in each turn of α-helix is:**
   (a) 2.8 (b) 3.2
   (c) 3.4 (d) 3.6
7. **In many proteins, the hydrogen bonding produces a regular coiled arrangement called:**
   (a) α-helix (b) β-helix
   (c) Both (a) and (b) (d) None of them
8. **The space covered by each amino acid residue of α-helix in nm is:**
   (a) 0.09 (b) 0.12
   (c) 0.15 (d) 0.18
9. **When egg albumin is coagulated (by heating):**
   (a) Only primary structure is changed
   (b) Only secondary structure is changed
   (c) Only tertiary structure is changed
   (d) Secondary and tertiary structure are changed
10. **Globulins are:**
    (a) Acidic proteins (b) Neutral proteins
    (c) Basic proteins (d) All of them
11. **In sickle cell anemia, a glutamic acid in β-chain is replaced by:**
    (a) Lysine (b) Leucine
    (c) Valine (d) Serine
12. **Precipitation or coagulation of proteins may be caused by:**
    (a) Heat (b) Change in pH
    (c) Heavy metal salts (d) All of them
13. **How much time do protein deficiency diseases take to develop?**
    (a) 7-15days (b) 15-20 days
    (c) 20-30 days (d) Months
14. **Can the adults live in a negative nitrogen balance for years?**
    (a) Yes (b) No
    (c) Sometimes (d) None of them
15. **Acidic amino acids amide:**
    (a) Asparagine (b) Serine
    (c) Leucine (d) None of them

16. Proline is:

(a) Imino acid
(b) Basic amino acid
(c) Acidic amino acid
(d) None of them

17. Amino acids on decarboxylation give:

(a) Amine
(b) Amide
(c) Ammonia
(d) All of them

18. Amino acids remain in:

(a) Ionized state
(b) Unionized state
(c) Either (a) or (b)
(d) Neither (a) or (b)

19. Irreversible precipitation of proteins caused by heating is known as:

(a) Polymerization
(b) Electrophoresis
(c) Denaturation
(d) Inversion

20. The linear arrangement of amino acid units in proteins is known as:

(a) Primary structure
(b) Secondary structure
(c) Tertiary structure
(d) Quaternary structure

21. The α-helix is a common form of:

(a) Primary structure
(b) Tertiary structure
(c) Secondary structure
(d) None of them

22. When glycine is heated it forms:

(a) Diketopiperazine
(b) Butyric acid
(c) Acrylic acid
(d) None of them

23. A zwitter ion has which of the following property:

(a) No net charge
(b) High melting point
(c) Solubility in water
(d) All of them

24. The amino acid found in protein structure is:

(a) Proline
(b) Leucine
(c) Lysine
(d) Glycine

25. Primary structure of protein is the sequence of amino acid in:

(a) Polypeptide
(b) R-group
(c) COOH group
(d) None of them

26. An example of phosphoprotein is:

(a) Casein
(b) Ferritin
(c) Hemoglobin
(d) None of them

27. Plasma contain........... % of proteins:

(a) 5.7% (b) 15-30%

(c) 50% (d) 20%

28. Which one of the following is non essential amino acid:

(a) Phenylalanine (b) Threonine

(c) Valine (d) Serine

29. During gestation total plasma proteins decrease due to an albumin decrease even though there is slight increase in:

(a) Fibrinogen (b) C-reactive proteins

(c) Globulins (d) None of them

30. The molecular weight of transferrin, a protein for iron transport is approximately:

(a) 1,40,000 Da (b) 76,000 Da

(c) 80,000 Da (d) 3,40,000 Da

31. For fractionation of serum proteins, which of the following methods can be used:

(a) Salt fractionation (b) Dye binding

(c) Colorimetric (d) All of them

32. In salt fractionation which one of the following is used most commonly:

(a) Sodium chloride (b) Ammonium sulphate

(c) Both (a) and (b) (d) None of them

33. Polypeptides with more than few hundred amino acid residues of ten fold into two or more stable globular units called:

(a) MOTIFS (b) Domains

(c) Both (a) and (b) (d) None of them

34. In ruminants plasma proteins are mixtures of:

(a) Glycoproteins (b) Conjugated proteins

(c) Lipoproteins (d) All of them

35. Amino acid containing Σ-amino group:

(a) Arginine (b) Tyrosine

(c) Histidine (d) Lysine

36. Distance travelled per turn of α-helix is:

(a) 0.36nm (b) 3.6nm

(c) 0.54nm (d) 0.15nm

37. Functional proteins include:

(a) Myosin
(b) Hemoglobin
(c) Cytochromes
(d) All of them

38. The decarboxylation product of tyrosine is:

(a) Glycine
(b) Alanine
(c) Tyramine
(d) Serine

39. Ammonium ion to the brain is:

(a) Beneficial
(b) Toxic
(c) Non-toxic
(d) No effect

40. The bonds in the protein structure which are not broken on denaturation:

(a) H-bond
(b) Ionic acid
(c) Peptide bond
(d) Disulphide bond

41. An intermediate of TCA cycle found in the reaction of urea cycle:

(a) Succinyl CoA
(b) Fumaric acid
(c) Oxalo acetate
(d) Isocitrate

42. The reaction given by two or more polypeptide linkages is:

(a) Biuret test
(b) Ninhydrin test
(c) Xanthoproteic test
(d) Pauley's test

43. The number of non essential amino acids is:

(a) 6
(b) 8
(c) 10
(d) 12

44. One of the following is a non-protein amino acid:

(a) Ornithine
(b) Homocysteine
(c) Histamine
(d) All of them

45. The amino acid required for the formation of glutathione:

(a) Glycine
(b) Cystine
(c) Epinephrine
(d) Thyroxine

46. The sequentor is an automatic machine to determine amino acid sequence in a polypeptide chain. The regent used in sequentor is:

(a) Sanger's reagent
(b) CNBR
(c) Trypsin
(d) Edman's reagent

47. Pick the acidic amino acid:

(a) Aspartic acid (b) Adenylic acid
(c) Arginine (d) Histidine

48. One of the following causes precipitation of proteins:

(a) Ammonium sulphate (b) Glycerol
(c) Creatinine (d) Urea

49. The amino acid that does not participate in transamination:

(a) Lysine (b) Glutamate
(c) Alanine (d) Tryptophan

50. Fibrous proteins have axial ratio of more than:

(a) 3 (b) 6
(c) 9 (d) 10 or more

51. Sulphur containing essential amino acid is:

(a) Methionine (b) Cysteine
(c) Cystine (d) None of them

52. Serum albumin has the molecular weight:

(a) 69000Da (b) 44000Da
(c) 1,50,000 Da (d) 6000Da

53. Functions of plasma proteins are:

(a) Nutritive (b) Transport
(c) Osmotic (d) All of them

54. Molecular weight of transferrin is:

(a) 56000 (b) 66000
(c) 76000 (d) None of them

55. In proteinuria urine contains:

(a) More plasma protein (b) Enzymes
(c) Both (a) and (b) (d) None of them

56. Membrane proteins:

(a) Catalyse chemical reactions (b) Mediate flow of nutrients
(c) Both (a) and (b) (d) None of them

57. The number of different amino acids found to be present in natural proteins are:

(a) 10 (b) 20

(c) 25 (d) 30

58. In many proteins, the hydrogen bonding produces a regular coiled arrangement called:

(a) α-Helix (b) β-Helix

(c) Both (a) and (b) (d) None of them

59. The digestibility of certain denatured proteins by proteolytic enzyme is:

(a) Increased (b) Decreased

(c) No change (d) All of them

60. Milk protein in the stomach of infants is digested by:

(a) Pepsin (b) Trypsin

(c) Chymotrypsin (d) Rennin

61. Which one of the following proteolytic enzyme is found mainly in infants?

(a) Pepsin (b) Trypsin

(c) Rennin (d) Chymotrypsin

62. In the small intestine, trypsin hydrolyses peptide linkages containing:

(a) Serine (b) Aspartate

(c) Arginine (d) Histidine

63. If one amino acid is fed in excess, the absorption of another is:

(a) Accelerated (b) Retarded

(c) Not affected (d) None of them

64. Absorption of the neutral amino acid requires:

(a) NAD^+ (b) $NADP^+$

(c) PLP (d) TPP

65. In uricotelic organisms, nitrogen of amino acids is removed as:

(a) Ammonia (b) Urea

(c) Uric acid (d) None of them

66. The unwanted amino acid abstracted from the tissues are either used up by tissue or in the liver converted into:

(a) Ammonia (b) Urea
(c) Ammonium salts (d) Uric acid

67. The building up and breaking down of protoplasm are concerned with the metabolism of:

(a) Carbohydrates (b) Fats
(c) Proteins (d) Minerals

68. Metabolism of all proteins ingested over and above the essential required is called:

(a) Endogenous metabolism (b) Exogenous metabolism
(c) Both (a) and (b) (d) None of them

69. The metabolism of protein is integrated with that of fat and carbohydrate through:

(a) Malate (b) Citrate
(c) Isocitrate (d) Oxaloacetate

70. The process of transamination requires:

(a) ATP (b) FAD
(c) NAD^+ (d) PLP

71. Transamination is a:

(a) Reversible process (b) Irreversible process
(c) Both (a) and (b) (d) None of them

72. The symptoms of ammonia poisoning include:

(a) Blurring of vision (b) Constipation
(c) Mental confusion (d) Diarrhoea

73. Synthesis of glutamine is accompanied by the hydrolysis of:

(a) ATP (b) ADP
(c) TPP (d) Creatinine phosphate

74. In brain, the major mechanism for removal of ammonia is the formation of:

(a) Glutamate (b) Aspartate
(c) Glutamine (d) Asparagine

75. The number of moles of ATP required in the synthesis of one mole of urea is:

(a) 1 (b) 2

(c) 3 (d) 4

76. The number of high energy bonds broken during the synthesis of one mole of urea is:

(a) 1 (b) 2

(c) 3 (d) 4

77. The number of amino acids involved during the synthesis of urea is:

(a) 3 (b) 4

(c) 5 (d) 6

78. How many grams of urea is excreted daily through urine in a normal individual?

(a) 10-20 (b) 15-25

(c) 20-30 (d) 25-35

79. Clinical symptoms in urea cycle disorder is:

(a) Diarrhoea (b) Oedema

(c) Drowsiness (d) Mental retardation

80. Which of the amino acid supplies methyl group for the biosynthesis of several physiologically important compounds?

(a) Glycine (b) Alanine

(c) Leucine (d) Methionine

81. Melanuria is caused by the abnormal catabolism of:

(a) Alanine (b) Tyrosine

(c) Proline (d) Tryptophan

82. Out of 200 different amino acids found in nature, the number of amino acids present in protein:

(a) 20 (b) 25

(c) 30 (d) 35

83. Enzyme catalysed hydrolysis of proteins produces amino acids of the form:

(a) D (b) DL

(c) L (d) All of them

84. The ionizable groups of amino acids are at least:

(a) 1 (b) 2

(c) 3 (d) 4

85. The carboxyl groups of amino acids exist almost entirely as the conjugated base at pH:

(a) 6.6 (b) 6.8

(c) 7.2 (d) 7.4

86. The pH of arginine is:

(a) 10.5 (b) 10.6

(c) 10.8 (d) 11.0

87. The neutral amino acid is:

(a) Leucine (b) Lysine

(c) Proline (d) Histidine

88. The amino acid containing hydroxyl group:

(a) Alanine (b) Isoleucine

(c) Arginine (d) Threonine

89. The basic amino acid:

(a) Glycine (b) Histidine

(c) Proline (d) Serine

90. The amino acid which synthesizes many hormones:

(a) Valine (b) Phenylalanine

(c) Alanine (d) Histidine

91. Amino acids are insoluble in:

(a) Acetic acid (b) Chloroform

(c) Ethanol (d) Benzene

92. The melting point of amino acids is above:

(a) 100°C (b) 180°C

(c) 200°C (d) 220°C

93. From two amino acids peptide bond formation involves removal of one mole of:

(a) Water (b) Ammonia

(c) Carbon dioxide (d) Carboxylic acid

94. Insulin degradation of disulphide bond formation is effected by:

(a) Pyruvate dehydrogenase (b) Xylitol reductase

(c) Glutathione reductase (d) Xanthine oxidase

95. The example of globulins:

(a) Leucosin (b) Tuberin

(c) Oryzenin (d) Legunelin

96. The example of scleroproteins:

(a) Glutenin (b) Gliadin

(c) Salmine (d) Elastin

97. The example of metalloprotein:

(a) Siderophilin (b) Osseomucoid

(c) Elastin (d) All of them

98. Protein structures are confirmed by weak bonds, the example of which is:

(a) Hydrophobic (b) Disulphide

(d) Peptide (d) All of them

99. Proteases produce polypeptides from proteins by:

(a) Oxidizing (b) Reducing

(c) Hydrolysing (d) None of them

100. Proteins react with biuret reagent which is suggestive of two or more:

(a) Hydrogen bonds (b) Peptide bonds

(c) Disulphide bonds (d) Hydrophobic bonds

101. Insulin is oxidized to separate the protein molecule into its constituent polypeptide chains without affecting the other part of the molecule by the use of:

(a) Performic acid (b) Oxalic acid

(c) Citric acid (d) Malic acid

102. The disulphide bond is not broken under the usual conditions of:

(a) Filtration (b) Reduction

(c) Oxidation (d) Denaturation

103. Each hydrogen bond is quite:

(a) Strong (b) Weak

(c) Both (a) and (b) (d) None of them

104. A coiled structure in which peptide bonds are folded in a regular manner by:

(a) Globular proteins (b) Fibrous proteins
(c) Both (a) and (b) (d) None of them

105. Many globular proteins are stable in solution although they lack in:

(a) Hydrogen bonds (b) Salt bonds
(c) Non-polar bonds (d) Disulphide bonds

106. α-helix is disrupted by certain amino acids like:

(a) Proline (b) Arginine
(c) Histidine (d) Lysine

107. α-helix is stabilized by:

(a) Hydrogen bonds (b) Disulphide bonds
(c) Salt bonds (d) Non-polar bonds

108. Glutamic dehydrogenase is a:

(a) Monomer (b) Tetramer
(c) Dimer (d) None of them

109. The hydrogen bonds between peptide linkages are interfered by:

(a) Guanidine (b) Uric acid
(c) Salicylic acid (d) Oxalic acid

110. The hydrogen bonds in the secondary and tertiary structure of proteins are directly attacked by:

(a) Salts (b) Alkalies
(c) Detergents (d) All of them

111. The digestibility of certain denatured proteins by proteolytic enzyme is:

(a) Decreased (b) Increased
(c) Normal (d) None of them

112. In case of severe denaturation of protein, there is:

(a) Reversible denaturation
(b) Moderate reversible denaturation
(c) Irreversible denaturation
(d) None of them

113. Bovine ribonuclease of single polypeptide chain of 124 amino acids residues with small molecular weight contains the number of disulphide bonds:

(a) 2 (b) 3
(c) 4 (d) 6

114. In glycoprotein, the carbohydrate is in the form of disaccharide units, the number of units are:

(a) 50-100 (b) 200-300
(c) 400-500 (d) 600-700

115. The disaccharide units of glycoproteins are attached to peptide chain, one per:

(a) 3.4 amino acid residues (b) 4.4 amino acid residues
(c) 5.4 amino acid residues (d) 6.4 amino acid residues

116. Chymotrypsin in the small intestine hydrolyses peptide linkage containing:

(a) Phenylalanine (b) Alanine
(c) Methionine (d) Valine

117. Carboxypeptidase B in the small intestine hydrolyses peptides containing:

(a) Leucine (b) Isoleucine
(c) Arginine (d) Cysteine

118. The transport of amino acids is regulated by active processes of different numbers:

(a) 1 (b) 2
(c) 3 (d) 4

119. The neutral amino acids for absorption need:

(a) TPP (b) B_6-PO_4
(c) NAD^+ (d) $NADP^+$

120. More than half of the protein of the liver and intestinal mucosa are broken down and resynthesized in:

(a) 10 days (b) 12 days
(c) 15 days (c) 18 days

121. The amino acids extracted from liver are not utilized for repair, but are broken down to:

(a) Ketoacids (b) Sulphur dioxide

(c) Water (d) Ammonia

122. Amino acids provide the nitrogen for the synthesis of:

(a) Bases of phospholipids (b) Uric acid

(c) Glycolipids (d) Chondroitin sulphates

123. Sulphur containing amino acids after catabolism produce a substance, which is excreted:

(a) SO_2 (b) HNO_3

(c) H_2SO_4 (d) H_3PO_4

124. Ethereal sulphate is synthesized from the amino acid:

(a) Neutral (b) Acidic

(c) Basic (d) Sulphur containing

125. Keratin, the protein of the hair is synthesized from the amino acid:

(a) Glycine (b) Serine

(c) Proline (d) Methionine

126. The transaminase activity needs the coenzyme:

(a) ATP (b) B_6-PO_4

(c) FAD^+ (d) NAD^+

127. Most amino acids are substrates for transamination except:

(a) Alanine (b) Threonine

(c) Serine (d) Valine

128. Oxidative conversions of many amino acids to their corresponding α-keto acids occur in mammalian:

(a) Liver and kidney (b) Adipose tissue

(c) Pancreas (d) Intestine

129. The α-keto acid is decarboxylated by H_2O_2 forming carboxylic acid with one carbon atom less in absence of the enzyme:

(a) Catalase (b) Decarboxylase

(c) Deaminase (d) Phosphatase

130. The activity of mammalian L-amino acid oxidase is quite:

(a) Slow (b) Rapid

(c) Both (a) and (b) (d) None of them

131. Ammonia intoxication symptoms occur when brain ammonia levels are:

(a) Slightly diminished (b) Highly diminished

(c) Increased (d) All of them

132. Ammonia production by the kidney is depressed in:

(a) Acidosis (b) Alkalosis

(c) Both (a) and (b) (d) None of them

133. Ammonia is excreted as ammonium salts during metabolic acidosis, but the majority is excreted as:

(a) Phosphates (b) Creatinine

(c) Uric acid (d) Urea

134. In bacteria, the synthesis of carbamoyl phosphate takes place from the substance:

(a) Ammonium salts (b) Ammonia

(c) Glutamine (d) Aspartate

135. The competitive inhibitor of arginine is:

(a) Citrulline (b) Malate

(c) Lysine (d) Serine

136. The biosynthesis of urea occurs mainly in:

(a) Cytosol (b) Mitochondria

(c) Microsomes (d) Nuclei

137. The sparing action of methionine is:

(a) Tyrosine (b) Cystine

(c) Arginine (d) Tryptophan

138. Following nitrogenous metabolites if present in excess in body fluids may exert toxic effects:

(a) Ammonia (b) Amino acid

(c) Porphyrin derivatives (d) All of them

139. NH_4^+ aminates glutamate to form glutamine requiring ATP and:

(a) Mg^{++} (b) Ca^{++}

(c) Na^+ (d) K^+

140. Glutathione is a:

(a) Dipeptide (b) Tripeptide

(c) Polypeptide (d) None of them

141. Glycine is synthesized from:

(a) Serine
(b) Choline
(c) Both (a) and (b)
(d) None of them

142. Hydroxyproline is converted to:

(a) Pyruvate
(b) Glyoxalate
(c) Both (a) and (b)
(d) None of them

143. For the formation of niacin from tryptophan, required vitamins are:

(a) B_2
(b) B_6
(c) Both (a) and (b)
(d) None of them

144. Leucine on catabolism yields:

(a) Acetoacetate
(b) Acetyl CoA
(c) Both (a) and (b)
(d) None of them

145. The activation of methionine requires:

(a) ATP
(b) Mg^{++}
(c) Glutathione
(d) All of them

146. By minor pathways, histidine is converted into:

(a) Carnosine
(b) Aniserine
(c) Both (a) and (b)
(d) None of them

147. Scleroproteins are similar to:

(a) Albumins
(b) Globulins
(c) Both (a) and (b)
(d) None of them

148. Antibody protein induced by immunization also undergo continual:

(a) Breakdown
(b) Synthesis
(c) Both (a) and (b)
(d) None of them

149. The globular proteins have the polypeptide chains of the type:

(a) Folded
(b) Coiled
(c) Both (a) and (b)
(d) None of them

150. Most fibrous proteins fulfill structural roles in:

(a) Skin
(b) Connective tissue
(c) Both (a) and (b)
(d) None of them

151. The amino acids obtained after hydrolysis of protein are separated and identified by:

(a) HPLC (b) Ion exchange

(c) Either of the two (d) Neither of the two

152. Disulphide bridges are disrupted by:

(a) Oxidizing agents (b) Reducing agents

(c) Both (a) and (b) (d) None of them

153. Acidic amino acids are the active agents in the process of:

(a) Deamination (b) Amination

(c) Both (a) and (b) (d) None of them

154. As a prosthetic group, transaminase requires a vitamin:

(a) B_1 (b) B_2

(c) B_6 (d) B_{12}

155. To the tissues, urea in higher concentration is:

(a) Useful (b) Partially useful

(c) Completely harmless (d) No effect

156. Hypervalinaemia is a condition in which valine accumulates in:

(a) Blood (b) Urine

(c) Both (a) and (b) (d) None of them

157. Histidine is catabolized by opening the ring to produce:

(a) Formiminoglutamic acid (b) Ornithine

(c) p-aminobenzoic acid (d) None of them

158. For the synthesis of collagen, the amino acid required are:

(a) Proline (b) Hydroxyproline

(c) Both (a) and (b) (d) None of them

159. The concentration of tryptophan in tissues is:

(a) Low (b) Very low

(c) High (d) Very high

160. A major pathway of tryptophan metabolism begins by opening 5-membered ring to form:

(a) Formyl kynurenine (b) Nicotinic acid

(c) 5-hydroxytryptamine (d) None of them

Answer Key

1	(b)	26	(a)	51	(a)	76	(d)
2	(a)	27	(a)	52	(a)	77	(d)
3	(a)	28	(d)	53	(d)	78	(c)
4	(d)	29	(c)	54	(a)	79	(d)
5	(b)	30	(b)	55	(c)	80	(d)
6	(d)	31	(a)	56	(c)	81	(b)
7	(a)	32	(b)	57	(b)	82	(a)
8	(c)	33	(b)	58	(a)	83	(c)
9	(d)	34	(a)	59	(a)	84	(b)
10	(b)	35	(d)	60	(d)	85	(d)
11	(c)	36	(c)	61	(c)	86	(c)
12	(d)	37	(d)	62	(c)	87	(a)
13	(d)	38	(c)	63	(b)	88	(d)
14	(a)	39	(d)	64	(c)	89	(b)
15	(a)	40	(c)	65	(c)	90	(b)
16	(a)	41	(b)	66	(b)	91	(d)
17	(a)	42	(a)	67	(c)	92	(c)
18	(a)	43	(c)	68	(b)	93	(a)
19	(c)	44	(a)	69	(d)	94	(c)
20	(c)	45	(a)	70	(d)	95	(b)
21	(c)	46	(d)	71	(a)	96	(d)
22	(c)	47	(a)	72	(c)	97	(a)
23	(a)	48	(a)	73	(a)	98	(a)
24	(a)	49	(c)	74	(c)	99	(c)
25	(a)	50	(d)	75	(c)	100	(b)

101	**(a)**	**116**	**(a)**	**131**	**(c)**	**146**	**(c)**
102	**(d)**	**117**	**(c)**	**132**	**(c)**	**147**	**(c)**
103	**(b)**	**118**	**(c)**	**133**	**(d)**	**148**	**(c)**
104	**(a)**	**119**	**(b)**	**134**	**(c)**	**149**	**(c)**
105	**(d)**	**120**	**(a)**	**135**	**(c)**	**150**	**(c)**
106	**(a)**	**121**	**(d)**	**136**	**(b)**	**151**	**(c)**
107	**(a)**	**122**	**(a)**	**137**	**(b)**	**152**	**(c)**
108	**(b)**	**123**	**(c)**	**138**	**(d)**	**153**	**(c)**
109	**(a)**	**124**	**(d)**	**139**	**(a)**	**154**	**(c)**
110	**(b)**	**125**	**(d)**	**140**	**(b)**	**155**	**(c)**
111	**(b)**	**126**	**(b)**	**141**	**(c)**	**156**	**(c)**
112	**(c)**	**127**	**(b)**	**142**	**(c)**	**157**	**(a)**
113	**(c)**	**128**	**(a)**	**143**	**(c)**	**158**	**(c)**
114	**(d)**	**129**	**(a)**	**144**	**(c)**	**159**	**(b)**
115	**(d)**	**130**	**(a)**	**145**	**(d)**	**160**	**(a)**

Chapter 5

Nucleic Acids and their Metabolism

1. **The three important units of DNA are:**
   (a) Bases, 2 de-oxyribose and phosphoric acid
   (b) Bases, ribose and phosphoric acid
   (c) Bases, 3 de-oxyribose and phosphoric acid
   (d) All the three

2. **Condensation product of adenine, ribose and phosphoric acid is named as:**
   (a) Adenosine (b) Adenylic acid
   (c) Adenine phosphate (d) None of them

3. **Thymine and deoxyribose form:**
   (a) Deoxycytidine (b) Deoxyadenosine
   (c) Deoxythymidine (d) Deoxyuridine

4. **The three common bases in DNA and RNA are:**
   (a) Adenine, guanine and cytosine (b) Adenine, guanine and uracil
   (c) Adenine, guanine and thymine (d) None of them

5. **The number of nucleotide units in a DNA molecule are:**
   (a) 800-4000 (b) 1000-6000
   (c) 1200-8000 (d) 1600-9000

6. The number of nucleotide pairs present in one turn of DNA is:

(a) 4 (b) 6

(c) 8 (d) 10

7. The number of hydrogen bonds present between the pair of guanosine nucleotide and cytosine nucleotide are:

(a) 1 (b) 2

(c) 3 (d) 4

8. DNA is denatured by:

(a) Heat (b) Acid

(c) Alkali (d) All of them

9. The number of nucleotide units in a RNA molecule is:

(a) 40 to 4000 (b) 50 to 5000

(c) 60 to 6000 (d) 70 to 7000

10. Unlike DNA, in RNA structure, the ratio of guanine to cytosine and adenine to uracil does not necessarily one since it is a:

(a) Double stranded molecule (b) Stable molecule

(c) Unstable molecule (d) Single stranded molecule

11. The number of nucleotides in a t-RNA molecule is:

(a) 70 (b) 75

(c) 80 (d) 85

12. Synthesis of RNA molecule is terminated by a signal which is recognized by:

(a) p(Rho) factor (b) δ-factor

(c) α-factor (d) None of them

13. The carbon atoms at position 4 and 5 and nitrogen atom at position 7 of purine base are supplied from:

(a) Valine (b) Alanine

(c) Glycine (d) Serine

14. The C_4, C_5 and C_6 and N_3 of pyrimidine base are derived from:

(a) Glutamic acid (b) Aspartic acid

(c) Glycine (d) Serine

15. The N_3 and N_9 of purine base are derived from the amide nitrogen of:

(a) Glutamate (b) Glutamine

(c) Asparagine (d) Aspartic acid

16. The end product of purine metabolism in other mammals except man is:

(a) Uric acid (b) Allantoin

(c) Ammonia (d) Creatinine

17. The net excretion of total uric acid in 24 hours in a normal man is:

(a) 100-300mg (b) 200-400mg

(c) 300-500mg (d) 400-600mg

18. A portion of uric acid is converted to urea and ammonia by intestinal:

(a) Urogenolysis (b) Ureolysis

(c) Uricolysis (d) Ureotolysis

19. The number of t-RNA molecules in every cell is at least:

(a) 10 (b) 15

(c) 20 (d) 25

20. Structural variation in cellular DNA do not affect key properties of DNA defined by Watson and Crick:

(a) Strand complementarity (b) Antiparallel strands

(c) Requirement of A=T and G≡C pairs (d) All of them

21. The PRPP synthase reaction is essential precursor for biosynthesis of:

(a) Purine nucleotide (b) Pyrimidine nucleotide

(c) Both (a) and (b) (d) None of them

22. Regulation of pyrimidine nucleotide biosynthesis involves control of:

(a) Gene expression (b) Enzyme activity

(c) Both (a) and (b) (d) None of them

23. On the DNA direction 5' to 3' polarity is followed by:

(a) DNA replication (b) RNA synthesis

(c) Protein synthesis (d) None of them

24. Pyrimidine catabolism does not yield:

(a) CO_2 (b) Uric acid

(c) NH_3 (d) β-amino isobutyrate

25. t-RNA molecules are more stable in:

(a) Eukaryotes (b) Bacteria

(c) Virus (d) Blue green algae

26. Inherited disorders of purine metabolism are due to the defective enzyme:

(a) Adenosine deaminase (b) Xanthine oxidase

(c) 5-phosphoribosyl-1-pyrophosphate (d) All of them

27. The two strands of double stranded helix are held together by:

(a) Hydrogen bond (b) Vanderwaal forces

(c) Hydrophobic bond (d) All of them

28. The second messenger obtained from ATP is:

(a) AMP (b) cAMP

(c) GAMP (d) None of them

29. Nucleotide and nucleic acid absorb UV light maximum at:

(a) 280mμ (b) 340mμ

(c) 260mμ (d) 300mμ

30. In gout defective enzyme is:

(a) Adenine phosphoribosyl transferase (b) PRPP synthase

(c) Xanthine oxidase (d) Adenosine deaminase

31. cAMP is formed from ATP by adenyl cyclase, which is activated by the hormone:

(a) Insulin (b) Epinephrine

(c) Testosterone (d) Progesterone

32. Which of the following nucleic acid base is found in mRNA but not in DNA?

(a) Adenine (b) Cytosine

(c) Guanine (d) Uracil

33. The following facts are true of all tRNA except that:

(a) 5'end phosphorylated (b) Are single chains

(c) Methylated based are found (d) Identical anticodon loop

34. Name the compound with greatest standard free energy:

(a) ATP (b) Phosphocreatine

(c) Cyclic AMP (d) Phosphoenol pyruvate

35. The backbone of nucleic acid structure is constructed by:

(a) Peptide bond (b) Glycosidic bond

(c) Phospho-diester linkage (d) All of them

36. Adenosine triphosphate has phosphate groups:

(a) 2 (b) 3

(c) 4 (d) 5

37. Which of the following pyrimidine base is found in RNA, but not in DNA?

(a) Adenine (b) Cytosine

(c) Guanine (d) Uracil

38. The double helical structure of DNA is held together by:

(a) Sulphur- sulphur linkage (b) Peptide linkage

(c) H-bonding (d) Glycosidic acid

39. Guanine is a:

(a) Pyrimidine (b) Purine

(c) Lipid (d) Protein

40. DNA and RNA contain:

(a) Adenine (b) Thymine

(c) Guanine (d) All of them

41. Nitrogen base not present in DNA structure:

(a) Adenine (b) Cytosine

(c) Guanine (d) Uracil

42. The nucleotide that serves as an intermediate for biosynthetic reactions:

(a) UDP-glucose (b) CPP-acylglycerol

(c) S-adenosylmethionine (d) All of them

43. Name the enzyme associated with hyperuricemia:

(a) PRPP synthetase (b) HGPRT

(c) Glucose-6-phosphatase (d) All of them

44. An enzyme of purine metabolism associated with immunodeficiency disease:

(a) Adenosine deaminase (b) Xanthine oxidase

(c) PRPP Synthetase (d) HGPRT

45. Orotic aciduria can be treated by diet rich in:

(a) Adenine (b) Guanine

(c) Uridine (d) Any one of them

46. The nitrogen atoms in the purine ring are obtained from:

(a) Glycine (b) Glutamine

(c) Aspartate (d) All of them

47. Nucleic acids are polymers of:

(a) Nucleosides (b) Nucleotides

(c) Both (a) and (b) (d) None of them

48. Under physiological conditions, DNA structure is pre-dominantly in:

(a) α-form (b) β-form

(c) Both (a) and (b) (d) None of them

49. Okazaki pieces are small fragments produced during:

(a) Replication (b) Transcription

(c) Translation (d) All of them

50. The powerful antagonists of folic acid action are:

(a) Aminopterin (b) Amethopterin

(c) Both (a) and (b) (d) None of them

51. In 1869 who defined what we now know to be nucleic acids:

(a) Chargaff (b) Davidson

(c) Miescher (d) Watson

52. Pyrimidine analogous include:

(a) 6-meraptopurine (b) 5-fluorouracil

(c) 8-azaguanine (d) Azaserine

53. As a rule of base pairing guanine links to:

(a) Thiamine (b) Uracil

(c) Either of the two (d) Neither of the two

54. If the double helix has not completely unwound, renaturation is very rapid when the temperature is:

(a) Lowered (b) Increased

(c) Remains same (d) None of them

55. Ribose-5-phosphate of nucleotides is synthesized in:

(a) Glycolytic pathway (b) HMP shunt pathway

(c) Both (a) and (b) (d) None of them

56. In their own synthesis, all purine nucleotides inhibit the:

(a) 1st Step (b) 2nd Step

(c) 3rd Step (d) None of them

57. The concentration of GPRT is normally highest in:

(a) Brain (b) Liver

(c) Kidney (d) None of them

58. Mononucleotides are acted upon by:

(a) Phosphatases (b) Pyrophosphorylase

(c) Both (a) and (b) (d) None of them

59. Purine analogous include:

(a) 6-mercaptopurine (b) 8-azaguanine

(c) Both (a) and (b) (d) None of them

60. The enzyme responsible for converting guanine to xanthine is known as:

(a) Guanase (b) Adenase

(c) Xanthine oxidase (d) None of them

61. The enzyme which converts adenine to hypoxanthine is known as:

(a) Adenase (b) Guanase

(c) Xanthine (d) None of them

62. The conversion of formylglycinamide ribonucleotide to formylglycinamidine ribonucleotide is accomplished by a reaction involving:

(a) L-Glutamine (b) ATP

(c) Both (a) and (b) (d) None of them

63. There are two pyrimidine derivatives which do not occur in the nucleic acids but which are of importance in the biosynthesis of the pyrimidines are:

(a) Orotic acid (b) Dihydro-orotic acid

(c) Both (a) and (b) (d) None of them

64. Nicotinamide adenine dinucleotide phosphate is the currently accepted name and abbreviation for:

(a) Triphosphopyridine nucleotide

(b) Triphosphopyrimidine nucleotide

(c) Both (a) and (b)

(d) None of them

65. The best role of purine and pyrimidine nucleotides is to serve as the monomeric precursors of:

(a) RNA
(b) DNA
(c) Both (a) and (b)
(d) None of them

66. The purine nucleotides act as the components of:

(a) FAD^+
(b) NAD^+
(c) $NADP^+$
(d) All of them

67. The pyrimidine nucleotides act as the high energy intermediates:

(a) UDPG
(b) ATP
(c) ADP
(d) AMP

68. The chemical name of thymine:

(a) 2,4-dioxypyrimidine
(b) 2-oxy-4-amino pyrimidine
(c) 2,4-dioxy-5-methyl pyrimidine
(d) None of them

69. The lactam form is the predominant tautomer of:

(a) Uracil
(b) Cytosine
(c) Adenine
(d) Xanthine

70. The chemical name 2-amino-6-oxypurine is said to be:

(a) Adenine
(b) Xanthine
(c) Guanine
(d) Hypoxanthine

71. N_7- methyl guanine has been found more recently in the nucleic acids of the cells of:

(a) Bacteria
(b) Yeast
(c) Plant
(d) Mammals

72. Hypoxanthine and ribose constitute:

(a) Adenosine
(b) Inosine
(c) Guanosine
(d) Cytidine

73. Thymine and deoxyribose form:

(a) Deoxycytidine
(b) Deoxyadenosine
(c) Deoxythymidine
(d) Deoxyuridine

74. The most abundant intracellular free nucleotide:

(a) ATP
(b) FAD^+
(c) NAD^+
(d) $NADP^+$

75. The intracellular cAMP concentration in μm are near:

(a) 3.0 (b) 2.0

(c) 1.0 (d) 0.5

76. The epimerization of galactose to glucose and vice-versa takes place by:

(a) UTP (b) CTP

(c) GTP (d) TPP

77. The biosynthesis of phosphoglycerides in animal tissues requires:

(a) ATP (b) CTP

(c) GTP (d) TPP

78. The chemical name 4-hydroxypyrazole pyrimidine is used for:

(a) Thioguanine (b) Mercaptopurine

(c) Azathiopurine (d) Allopurinol

79. The "transforming factor" is used for the name of:

(a) RNA (b) DNA

(c) tRNA (d) None of them

80. The double stranded DNA molecule loses its viscosity upon:

(a) Denaturation (b) Filtration

(c) Sedimentation (d) Concentration

81. Within the single turn of DNA the number of base pair exists:

(a) 4 (b) 6

(c) 8 (d) 10

82. Each turn of the DNA structure has a pitch in nm of:

(a) 1.4 (b) 2.4

(c) 3.4 (d) 4.4

83. Chromatin contains the number of repeating units in nm:

(a) 10 (b) 15

(c) 20 (d) 25

84. The concentration of ATP in living mammalian cells in m mole is near:

(a) 0.2 (b) 0.4

(c) 0.6 (d) 1.0

85. Messenger RNA has a molecular weight of:

(a) 15000-30000 (b) 20000-35000

(c) 25000-40000 (d) 30000-50000

86. Of the total cellular RNA molecules the per cent of transfer RNA molecules amounts to:

(a) 5-10 (b) 8-16

(c) 10-20 (d) 15-30

87. All tRNA molecules have a common CCA sequence at the:

(a) 3' termini (b) 5'-termini

(c) 3',5'- termini (d) All of them

88. In nearly all tRNA molecules, there is a loop containing the nucleotides of:

(a) Pseudouridine (b) Ribothymine

(c) Both (a) and (b) (d) None of them

89. In tRNA molecules, there is another loop containing minor base:

(a) Uracil (b) Dihydrouracil

(c) Cytosine (d) Dihydrocytosine

90. The per cent of ribosomal RNA of RNA within the cell is:

(a) 60 (b) 70

(c) 80 (d) 90

91. Gene is a segment of DNA molecule containing base pairs about:

(a) 300 (b) 400

(c) 500 (d) 600

92. The fragments of DNA attached RNA initiator component were discovered by:

(a) Watson and Crick (b) Okazaki

(c) Peterson (d) Nelson

93. The promoter site at which the synthesis of new RNA molecule begins with the help of another factor:

(a) σ (b) γ

(c) β (d) α

94. The binding of prokaryotic DNA-dependent RNA polymerase to promoter sites of genes is inhibited by the antibiotic:

(a) Septran (b) Streptomycin

(c) Aureomycin (d) Rifampin

95. 5-phosphoribosylamine reacts with glycine to produce glycinamide ribosyl phosphate by glycinamide kinosynthetase in presence of:

(a) ATP (b) GTP

(c) UTP (d) CTP

96. Origin of urinary uric acid is:

(a) Exogenous (b) Endogenous

(c) Both (a) and (b) (d) None of them

97. Blood uric acid level increases in:

(a) Hemolytic anemia (b) Thalassemia

(c) Both (a) and (b) (d) None of them

98. Chemotherapy of cancer and viral infections involves the use of:

(a) Cytarabine (b) Vidarabine

(c) Both (a) and (b) (d) None of them

99. In size and stability, the messenger RNA is:

(a) Homogenous (b) Heterogenous

(c) Both (a) and (b) (d) None of them

100. Nucleoproteins are conjugated proteins containing basic protein:

(a) Protamine (b) Histones

(c) Either of the two (d) Neither of the two

101. The complete ribosome contains two sites on mRNA:

(a) P site (b) A site

(c) Both (a) and (b) (d) None of them

102. When a pair carries genes with the same tallness, individual is said to be:

(a) Heterozygous (b) Homozygous

(c) Either (a) or (b) (d) Neither (a) or (b)

103. When one of the pair tallness and the other gene shortness, individual is:

(a) Heterozygous (b) Homozygous

(c) Either (a) or (b) (d) Neither (a) or (b)

104. Many effective antibiotics interact with the proteins of prokaryotic ribosomes and thus protein synthesis is:

(a) Inhibited
(b) Promoted
(c) Remains stationary
(d) None of them

105. The formation of one peptide bond causes the hydrolysis of two molecules of:

(a) ATP
(b) GTP
(c) Both (a) and (b)
(d) None of them

106. The adapter molecules translating the code words into the amino acid sequence are the:

(a) tRNA
(b) mRNA
(c) rRNA
(d) All of them

107. The end product of nitrogen catabolism in uricotelic animals is:

(a) Urea
(b) Uric acid
(c) Ammonia
(d) All of them

108. The protein part of nucleoproteins is easily hydrolyzed by:

(a) Intestinal enzymes
(b) Gastric enzymes
(c) Both (a) and (b)
(d) None of them

109. Adenine nucleotides centrally involved in cellular metabolism:

(a) AMP
(b) ADP
(c) ATP
(d) All of them

110. Body has got the capability of synthesizing purines and pyrimidines from the product of:

(a) Carbohydrate metabolism
(b) Protein metabolism
(c) Both (a) and (b)
(d) None of them

Answer Key

1	(a)	26	(a)	51	(c)	76	(a)
2	(b)	27	(d)	52	(b)	77	(b)
3	(c)	28	(b)	53	(c)	78	(d)
4	(a)	29	(a)	54	(a)	79	(d)
5	(d)	30	(c)	55	(b)	80	(a)
6	(d)	31	(b)	56	(a)	81	(d)
7	(c)	32	(d)	57	(a)	82	(c)
8	(d)	33	(a)	58	(c)	83	(a)
9	(c)	34	(a)	59	(c)	84	(d)
10	(d)	35	(c)	60	(a)	85	(d)
11	(b)	36	(b)	61	(a)	86	(c)
12	(a)	37	(d)	62	(c)	87	(a)
13	(c)	38	(a)	63	(c)	88	(c)
14	(b)	39	(b)	64	(a)	89	(b)
15	(b)	40	(d)	65	(c)	90	(c)
16	(b)	41	(d)	66	(d)	91	(d)
17	(d)	42	(d)	67	(a)	92	(b)
18	(c)	43	(d)	68	(c)	93	(d)
19	(c)	44	(a)	69	(a)	94	(d)
20	(c)	45	(c)	70	(c)	95	(a)
21	(a)	46	(d)	71	(d)	96	(c)
22	(b)	47	(b)	72	(b)	97	(c)
23	(a)	48	(a)	73	(c)	98	(c)
24	(b)	49	(a)	74	(a)	99	(b)
25	(b)	50	(c)	75	(c)	100	(c)

101	**(c)**	**104**	**(a)**	**107**	**(b)**	**110**	**(c)**
102	**(b)**	**105**	**(c)**	**108**	**(c)**		
103	**(a)**	**106**	**(a)**	**109**	**(d)**		

Chapter 6

Inorganic Elements and their Metabolism

1. **Elements required to be present in diet in amounts more than 1mg are called:**
   (a) Macro-elements (b) Micro-elements
   (c) Semi-microelements (d) None of them

2. **Which one of the following is an essential element?**
   (a) Arsenic (b) Silicon
   (c) Copper (d) Aluminium

3. **The number of principal mineral elements are:**
   (a) 5 (b) 6
   (c) 7 (d) 8

4. **The most important dietary source of calcium is:**
   (a) Egg yolk (b) Cauliflower
   (c) Milk (d) Meat

5. **The absorption of calcium is increased by the dietary high levels of:**
   (a) Cereals (b) Fats
   (c) Proteins (d) Vitamin A

6. **Calcium absorption is interfered by:**
   (a) Phytic acid (b) Fatty acids
   (c) Oxalic acid (d) All of them

7. **Calcium is found in bones in the form of:**
   (a) $CaCO_3$ (b) $Ca_3 (PO_4)_2$
   (c) $C_aCO_{3.}nCa_3 (PO_4)_2$ (d) $Ca (C_2O_4)_2$

8. **In plasma, calcium exists in how many forms of physiological different forms:**
   (a) 1 (b) 2
   (c) 3 (d) 4

9. **The percentage of calcium in mg in non-ionized form is about:**
   (a) 3 (b) 4
   (c) 5 (d) 6

10. **Calcium is required for the activation of:**
    (a) Isocitrate dehydrogenase (b) ATPase
    (c) Fumarase (d) Succinate thiokinase

11. **Calcium is excreted through:**
    (a) Urine (b) Feces
    (c) Sweat (d) All of them

12. **The concentration of serum calcium may drop below 7mg/100ml in:**
    (a) Rickets (b) Tetany
    (c) Hypoparathyroidism (d) Hyperparathyroidism

13. **Phosphorus contributes about:**
    (a) 0.01% of total body weight (b) 0.1% of total body weight
    (c) 1% of total body weight (d) 10% of total body weight

14. **Bones and teeth are rich in:**
    (a) Inorganic form of phosphorus (b) Organic form of phosphorus
    (c) Both (a) and (b) (d) None of them

15. **In the body, magnesium acts as antagonist of:**
    (a) Sodium (b) Potassium
    (c) Calcium (d) None of them

16. Sodium and potassium are the main:

(a) Intracellular cations

(b) Extracellular cations

(c) Intracellular and extracellular, respectively

(d) Extracellular and intracellular, respectively

17. The highest concentration of chloride ions is found in:

(a) Whole blood (b) Plasma

(c) CSF (d) Nerves

18. Which of the following plays dominant role in maintaining the normal osmotic pressure of the different body fluids:

(a) Na^+ (b) K^+

(c) Cl^- (d) All the three

19. Which of the following plays dominant role in transporting CO_2 in the body?

(a) Na^+ (b) K^+

(c) Cl^- (d) All the three

20. Which of the following forms of iron is better absorbed?

(a) Fe^{2+} (b) Fe^{3+}

(c) Both equal (d) None of them

21. Which of the following elements is required for the development of erythrocytes?

(a) Calcium (b) Magnesium

(c) Iron (d) Potassium

22. Wilson's disease is associated with the abnormal metabolism of:

(a) Iron (b) Potassium

(c) Iodine (d) Copper

23. Hemoglobin formation needs both:

(a) Iron and zinc (b) Iron and calcium

(c) Iron and copper (d) Iron and magnesium

24. Zinc is a constituent of:

(a) Aldolase (b) Amylase

(c) Malate dehydrogenase (d) Carbonic anhydrase

25. Deficiency of cobalt results in:

(a) Anemia
(b) Diabetes
(c) Headache
(d) None of them

26. Dental fluorosis is characterized by:

(a) Low intake of fluorine
(b) Excess intake of fluorine
(c) Neither of the two
(d) Both (a) and (b)

27. The amount of water excreted in feces is:

(a) 90ml/day
(b) 95ml/day
(c) 100ml/day
(d) 105ml/day

28. Dehydration may be ordinarily corrected by parenteral ingestion of solution of:

(a) NaCl
(b) $ZnCl_2$
(c) $MgCl_2$
(d) $CaCl_2$

29. Dehydration is a problem as regards to:

(a) Vomiting
(b) Typhoid
(c) Uremia
(d) Hot climate

30. The volume of CSF in a normal adult is:

(a) 30-50ml
(b) 100-150ml
(c) 180-200ml
(d) 250-300ml

31. The mitochondrial superoxide dismutase contains:

(a) Mg^{2+}
(b) Mn^{2+}
(c) Zn^{2+}
(d) Co^{2+}

32. Oxidases are conjugated proteins having the prosthetic group:

(a) Mg
(b) Mn
(c) Cu
(d) Fe

33. Phenolase is an enzyme containing:

(a) Cu
(b) Co
(c) Fe
(d) Zn

34. The following element is involved in wound healing:

(a) Calcium
(b) Sodium
(c) Zinc
(d) Magnesium

35. Calcium absorption is favoured by:

(a) Low pH (b) High pH

(c) Neutral pH (d) None of them

36. Calcium absorption is facilitated by the amino acid:

(a) Lysine (b) Arginine

(c) Both (a) and (b) (d) None of them

37. Magnesium deficiency causes:

(a) Neuromuscular irritation (b) Weakness

(c) Convulsion (d) All of them

38. When serum sodium level falls below normal, condition is:

(a) Hyponatremia (b) Hypernatremia

(c) Both (a) and (b) (d) None of them

39. The symptoms of hypernatremia include:

(a) Increase in blood volume (b) Hypertension

(c) Both (a) and (b) (d) None of them

40. Principal intracellular cation is:

(a) Potassium (b) Sodium

(c) Magnesium (d) None of them

41. Potassium is required for the:

(a) Transmission of nerve impulse

(b) Biosynthesis of proteins by ribosomes

(c) Both (a) and (b)

(d) None of them

42. Cushing syndrome is:

(a) Over activity of adrenal cortex (b) Adrenocortical insufficiency

(c) Both (a) and (b) (d) None of them

43. Addison's disease is:

(a) Over activity of adrenal cortex (b) Adrenocortical insufficiency

(c) Both (a) and (b) (d) None of them

44. Chloride is involved in the regulation of:

(a) Acid-base equilibrium (b) Fluid balance

(c) Osmotic pressure (d) All of them

45. An increase in serum chloride concentration may be due to:

(a) Dehydration (b) Respiratory acidosis

(c) Cushing syndrome (d) All of them

46. Iron absorption is diminished by:

(a) Copper deficiency (b) Administration of alkali

(c) Both (a) and (b) (d) None of them

47. In hemochromatosis, iron is deposited in:

(a) Liver (b) Spleen

(c) Pancreas (d) All of them

48. The symptoms of Menke's disease include:

(a) Decreased copper in plasma (b) Anemia

(c) Depigmentation of hair (d) All of them

49. Manganese is required for the:

(a) Formation of bone (b) Proper reproduction

(c) Normal functioning of nervous system (d) All of them

50. Molybdenum is a constituent of the enzyme:

(a) Xanthine oxidase (b) Aldehyde oxidase

(c) Sulfite oxidase (d) None of them

51. Cobalt content of vitamin B_{12} is:

(a) 4% by weight (b) 6% by weight

(c) 7% by weight (d) 8% by weight

52. Manifestations of molybdenosis include:

(a) Impairment in growth (b) Diarrhoea

(c) Anemia (d) All of them

53. Selenium along with vitamin E prevents the development of:

(a) Hepatic necrosis (b) Muscular dystrophy

(c) Both (a) and (b) (d) None of them

54. Chromium deficiency causes disturbance in the metabolism of:

(a) Carbohydrate (b) Protein

(c) Lipid (d) All of them

55. Chromium decreases in:

(a) Serum LDL
(b) Serum HDL
(c) Serum VLDL
(d) None of them

56. Manifestations of selenosis include:

(a) Weight loss
(b) Emotional disturbances
(c) Garlic odor in breath
(d) All of them

57. Which of the following should be added regularly in traces of drinking water so as to avoid dental caries?

(a) Chlorine
(b) Fluorine
(c) Bromine
(d) Iodine

58. What percentage of total calcium of the body is found in bones?

(a) 39
(b) 59
(c) 79
(d) 99

59. Forms of calcium recognized in plasma:

(a) Ionized
(b) Diffusible
(c) Non-diffusible
(d) All of them

60. The ionizable fraction of calcium participates in:

(a) Blood coagulation
(b) Neuromuscular activity
(c) Myocardial activity
(d) All of them

61. Phytic acid found in cereal grains forms insoluble salts with:

(a) Ca^{++}
(b) Mg^{++}
(c) Both (a) and (b)
(d) None of them

62. Concentration of potassium per kg muscle is about:

(a) 3.2g
(b) 4.2g
(c) 5.2g
(d) 6.2g

63. Insufficient sodium intake can give rise to heat stroke, which is characterized by:

(a) Muscular weakness
(b) Nausea
(c) Fever
(d) All of them

64. Foods of vegetable origin are richer in:

(a) Sodium
(b) Potassium
(c) Calcium
(d) Magnesium

65. The metabolism of chlorine cannot be separated from the metabolism of:

(a) Calcium (b) Magnesium
(c) Potassium (d) Sodium

66. Major portion of iodine remains confined to the:

(a) Thyroid gland (b) Prostate gland
(c) Lungs (d) Thymus

67. Fluorine is present in various tissues of body, particularly in:

(a) Bone (b) Teeth
(c) Both (a) and (b) (d) None of them

68. What is the percentage of fluorine present in a normal bone:

(a) 0.01-0.03 (b) 0.03-0.08
(c) 0.08-0.12 (d) 0.12-0.18

69. What is the percentage of fluorine present in dental enamel:

(a) 0.04-0.08 (b) 0.01-0.02
(c) 0.08-0.12 (d) 0.10-0.15

70. Resorption of skeletal calcium is excreted by:

(a) Pregnancy (b) Lactation
(c) Both (a) and (b) (d) None of them

71. Zinc is a component of active:

(a) Insulin (b) Progesterone
(c) Prolactin (d) Protamines

72. The chief storage sites for manganese in the body are:

(a) Kidney (b) Liver
(c) Both (a) and (b) (d) None of them

73. Manganese is involved in activating the enzyme:

(a) Peptidase (b) Carboxylase
(c) Cholinesterase (d) All of them

74. The half life of plasma iron is about:

(a) 90 minutes (b) 70 minutes
(c) 50 minutes (d) 30 minutes

75. The efficiency of iron absorption can greatly increase in:
(a) Pregnancy
(b) Iron deficiency
(c) Most kinds of anemia
(d) All of them

76. The important storage organs of iron are:
(a) Liver
(b) Spleen
(c) Red marrow
(d) All of them

77. Molybdenum is rapidly and effectively absorbed in human beings by:
(a) Liver
(b) Kidney
(c) Intestinal tract
(d) Pancreas

78. Genetic disturbances of copper metabolism:
(a) Hepato lenticular degeneration
(b) Wilson's disease
(c) Either of the two
(d) Neither of the two

79. In heart failure, which mitochondrial ions are depleted?
(a) Sodium
(b) Potassium
(c) Calcium
(d) Magnesium

80. In most of the cases, hyperkalemia results on account of the:
(a) Liver failure
(b) Pancreas failure
(c) Renal failure
(d) Tumors in the bones

81. Cushing's syndrome may be diagnosed by:
(a) Hypokalemia
(b) Hyponatremia
(c) Hypocalcemia
(d) Hypoglycemia

82. Loss of mineral mass is seen in all except:
(a) Gluco-corticoid therapy
(b) Hypoparathyroidism
(c) Immobilization
(d) None of them

83. The non-heme iron is completely protein bound, which exists in the form of:
(a) Storage
(b) Transport
(c) Both (a) and (b)
(d) None of them

84. Sulphur is present primarily in the cell protein in the form of:
(a) Cysteine
(b) Methionine
(c) Both (a) and (b)
(d) None of them

85. Anemia is due to the deficiency in:

(a) Sodium (b) Potassium

(c) Phosphorus (d) Iron

86. Serum phosphate concentration is 1-2mg/100ml in:

(a) Rickets (b) Tetany

(c) Osteoporosis (d) Hyperthyroidism

87. Prolonged hypokalemia causes injury to:

(a) Myocardium (b) Kidneys

(c) Both (a) and (b) (d) None of them

88. Hypernatremia occurs in prolonged treatment of:

(a) Cortisone (b) ACTH

(c) Both (a) and (b) (d) None of them

89. The daily loss of calcium in mg in sweat is about:

(a) 12 (b) 13

(c) 14 (d) 15

90. The percentage of calcium excreted in feces is:

(a) 40 to 60 (b) 50 to 70

(c) 60 to 80 (d) 70 to 90

91. Calcium in the complex form is about:

(a) 8mg % (b) 6mg %

(c) 4mg % (d) 2mg %

92. Calcium absorption is interfered by:

(a) Fatty acids (b) Amino acids

(c) Vitamin D (d) Vitamin B_{12}

93. Cobalt is a constituent of:

(a) Folic acid (b) Vitamin B_{12}

(c) Niacin (d) Biotin

94. Zinc is a constituent of:

(a) Carbonic anhydrase (b) Maltase dehydrogenase

(c) Aldolase (d) Amylase

95. The essential trace elements include:

(a) Lead (b) Nickel

(c) Boron (d) Cobalt

96. The trace elements are subdivided into:

(a) Two groups (b) Three groups

(c) Four groups (d) None of them

97. The principal mineral elements are also said to be:

(a) Macronutrients (b) Micronutrients

(c) Semi-micronutrients (d) None of them

98. How much percentage of total iron of human body does remain in hemoglobin:

(a) 25 (b) 50

(c) 75 (d) More than 75

99. Excretion of molybdenum in humans is primarily by way of the:

(a) Urine (b) Feces

(c) Sweat (d) Tears

100. Among the elements needed in quantities greater than 1mg for human beings are:

(a) Calcium (b) Copper

(c) Zinc (d) Nickel

Answer Key

1	(a)	26	(b)	51	(a)	76	(d)
2	(c)	27	(c)	52	(d)	77	(c)
3	(c)	28	(a)	53	(c)	78	(c)
4	(c)	29	(c)	54	(d)	79	(b)
5	(c)	30	(d)	55	(a)	80	(c)
6	(d)	31	(b)	56	(d)	81	(a)
7	(c)	32	(c)	57	(b)	82	(b)
8	(c)	33	(a)	58	(d)	83	(c)
9	(c)	34	(c)	59	(d)	84	(c)
10	(b)	35	(a)	60	(d)	85	(d)
11	(d)	36	(c)	61	(c)	86	(a)
12	(c)	37	(d)	62	(a)	87	(c)
13	(d)	38	(a)	63	(d)	88	(c)
14	(a)	39	(c)	64	(b)	89	(d)
15	(c)	40	(a)	65	(d)	90	(d)
16	(d)	41	(c)	66	(a)	91	(d)
17	(c)	42	(a)	67	(c)	92	(a)
18	(a)	43	(b)	68	(a)	93	(b)
19	(c)	44	(d)	69	(b)	94	(a)
20	(a)	45	(d)	70	(c)	95	(d)
21	(c)	46	(c)	71	(a)	96	(b)
22	(d)	47	(d)	72	(c)	97	(a)
23	(c)	48	(d)	73	(d)	98	(c)
24	(d)	49	(d)	74	(a)	99	(a)
25	(a)	50	(d)	75	(d)	100	(a)

Chapter 7

Enzymes

1. **An example of extracellular enzyme is:**
   (a) Glucokinase (b) Hexokinase
   (c) Glucose-6-phosphatase (d) Pepsin

2. **Pepsin is the active enzyme of the pre-enzyme:**
   (a) Pepsinogen (b) Trypsinogen
   (c) Chymotrypsinogen (d) None of them

3. **The protein moiety of an enzyme is known as:**
   (a) Holoenzyme (b) Apoenzyme
   (c) Coenzyme (d) None of them

4. **Co-enzyme involved in hydrogen transfer is:**
   (a) Thiamine pyrophosphate (b) Co-enzyme A
   (c) ATP (d) FAD

5. **The optimum temperature of an enzyme of human body is:**
   (a) 22°C (b) 25°C
   (c) 37°C (d) 47°C

6. **The group transferring coenzyme is:**
   (a) DPN (b) TPN
   (c) FAD^+ (d) CoA

7. **Oxidases are generally inhibited by:**
   (a) Cyanides (b) Fluorides
   (c) Salts of mercury (d) Salt of silver

8. **The enzyme lysozyme is used in the treatment of:**
   (a) Coronary disease (b) Liver disease
   (c) Leukaemia (d) Eye disease

9. **The enzyme which acts on single hydrogen donor with incorporation of oxygen is:**
   (a) Succinate thiokinase (b) Glycogen synthase
   (c) Trptophan oxygenase (d) Urease

10. **Lactate dehyrogenase exists in:**
    (a) 2 isozymic forms (b) 3 isozymic forms
    (c) 4 isozymic forms (d) 5 isozymic forms

11. **Nicotinamide is the active component of:**
    (a) DPN (b) TPN
    (c) Both (a) and (b) (d) None of them

12. **For the enzymes best preservative is:**
    (a) Toluene (b) Benzene
    (c) Hexane (d) None of them

13. **Enzymes that catalyze removal of groups from substrates without addition or removal of water are called:**
    (a) Lyases (b) Synthetases
    (c) Both (a) and (b) (d) None of them

14. **Enzymes which remove hydrogen from the substrate and pass it directly to oxygen are known:**
    (a) Oxygenases (b) Oxidases
    (c) Aerobic dehydrogenases (d) Anaerobic dehydrogenases

15. **Oxidases are the conjugated proteins having the prosthetic group:**
    (a) Magnesium (b) Manganese
    (c) Copper (d) Iron

16. **Aerobic dehydrogenases have the prosthetic group:**
    (a) ATP (b) NAD^+
    (c) FAD^+ (d) $NADP^+$

17. Many enzymes require for their maximal activity:

(a) Metallic ions (b) Vitamins

(c) Hormones (d) None of them

18. Freezing of enzyme results in:

(a) Concentration of salt (b) Concentration of enzyme

(c) Both (a) and (b) (d) None of them

19. AST found in:

(a) Cytosol (b) Mitochondria

(c) Both (a) and (b) (d) None of them

20. In plasma enzymes are elevated in:

(a) Cell damage (b) Enzyme induction

(c) Both (a) and (b) (d) None of them

21. Amount of any single enzyme in serum is a function of its:

(a) Concentration in cells (b) Total tissue mass

(c) Both (a) and (b) (d) None of them

22. In most instances serum enzyme determinations are utilized as screening test to detect organ involvement, most desirable are:

(a) High sensitivity (b) Reasonable specificity

(c) Both (a) and (b) (d) None of them

23. The non-protein part of holoenzyme is:

(a) Co-enzyme (b) Cofactor

(c) Both (a) and (b) (d) None of them

24. Phosphofructokinase is allosterically activated by:

(a) AMP (b) ADP

(c) Both (a) and (b) (d) None of them

25. The enzymes loose the activity above:

(a) 70°C (b) 60°C

(c) 90°C (d) 100°C

26. Alcohol dehydrogenase from liver contains:

(a) Sodium (b) Potassium

(c) Zinc (d) Copper

27. Enzymes are usually named by adding suffix- ase to the main part of name of substrate on which they act except:

(a) Erepsin (b) Maltase
(c) Lactase (d) Sucrase

28. Some enzymes are named by their functions only *e.g.*:

(a) Ptyalin (b) Pepsin
(c) Reductase (d) Trypsin

29. Some enzymes acting on the substrates are freely described by the adjectives *e.g.*:

(a) Lactate dehydrogenase (b) Lipolytic
(c) Cytochrome oxidase (d) Phosphatase

30. The enzyme which uses oxygen as hydrogen acceptor *e.g.*:

(a) Tyrosinase (b) Succinate dehydrogenase
(c) Aconitase (d) Carboxylase

31. The enzyme which uses H_2O_2 as substrate *e.g.*:

(a) Catalase (b) Malate dehydrogenase
(c) Ascorbic oxidase (d) Phosphorylase

32. The enzyme which acts on paired donors with incorporation of oxygen into one donor:

(a) Pyruvate kinase (b) Enolase
(c) Steroid hydroxylase (d) Glycerokinase

33. The enzyme acting on peptide bonds:

(a) Hexokinase (b) Chymotrypsin
(c) SGOT (d) Glucose-6-phosphatase

34. Enzyme exergonic reaction means the system undergoes a loss of free energy:

(a) Synthetase (b) Phosphatase
(c) Hexokinase (d) Urease

35. The maximum activity of most of the enzymes is at the optimum pH:

(a) Between 2 and 3 (b) Between 4 and 5
(c) Between 5 and 9 (d) Between 7 and 12

36. The peroxidase has the coenzyme:

(a) FAD^+ (b) NAD^+
(c) $NADP^+$ (d) None of them

37. Enzymes of digestive tract are:

(a) Extracellular (b) Intracellular

(c) Both (a) and (b) (d) None of them

38. The enzyme containing an aromatic hetero-ring in the structure:

(a) Biotin (b) TPP

(c) Sugar phosphate (d) Coenzyme Q

39. The example of hydrogen transferring coenzyme:

(a) B6-PO_4 (b) $NADP^+$

(c) TPP (d) ATP

40. A dipeptide can be attacked by the number of enzymes:

(a) One (b) Two

(c) Three (d) Four

41. The isocitrate dehydrogenase reaction is analogues to:

(a) Pyruvate dehydrogenase (b) Lactate dehydrogenase

(c) 6-phosphogluconate dehydrogenase (d) None of them

42. Trypsin of pancreatic juice is a mixture of:

(a) Trypsin (b) Chymotrypsin A

(c) Chymotrypsin B (d) All of them

43. The loss of enzyme activity by oxidation may be regained by:

(a) Cysteine (b) Glutathione

(c) Either of the two (d) Neither of two

44. Coenzyme functioning as hydrogen acceptor in dehydrogenation reaction are:

(a) NAD^+ (b) $NADP^+$

(c) Both (a) and (b) (d) None of them

45. The enzymes that occur in a number of different forms and differ each other chemically, electrophoretically and immunologically are called:

(a) Isoenzymes (b) Antienzymes

(c) Co-enzymes (d) None of them

46. Maltase catalyzes the hydrolysis of:

(a) α-glycosides (b) β-glycosides

(c) Both (a) and (b) (d) None of them

47. Selenium containing enzyme is:

(a) Glutathione peroxidase
(b) Xanthine oxidase
(c) Both (a) and (b)
(d) None of them

48. In competitive inhibition:

(a) Apparent Km unchanged
(b) Apparent Km decreased
(c) Vmax decreased
(d) Vmax unchanged

49. Di-isopropyl fluorophosphates (DFP) react with serine proteases stoichiometrically and irreversibly and therefore is a:

(a) Competitive inhibitor
(b) Non-competitive inhibitor
(c) Uncompetitive inhibitor
(d) Allosteric inhibitor

50. Which of the following is not a component of coenzyme A?

(a) Adenylic acid
(b) Pantothenic acid
(c) Cysteamine
(d) Acetic acid

51. As a coenzyme pyruvate decarboxylase requires:

(a) Coenzyme A
(b) NAD^+
(c) FMN
(d) Thiamine pyrophosphate

52. An enzyme of saliva that hydrolyzes starch is:

(a) Pepsin
(b) β-amylase
(c) Lysozyme
(d) α-Amylase

53. All the following gastro-intestinal enzymes are secreted as inactive zymogens (proenzymes) except:

(a) Ribonuclease
(b) Trypsin
(c) Chymotrypsin
(d) Carboxypeptidase

54. Which enzyme has the greatest specificity for peptide bonds on the carboxyl side of a cationic amino acid side chain:

(a) Carboxypeptidase
(b) Trypsin
(c) Rennin
(d) Chymotrypsin

55. In non-competitive inhibition:

(a) Concentration of active enzyme molecule reduced
(b) Vmax increased
(c) Concentration of active enzyme molecule unchanged
(d) Km increased

56. Dehydrogenases use as coenzymes all of the following except:

(a) NAD^+
(b) $NADP^+$
(c) FAD
(d) Ferriprotoporphyrin

57. In an enzyme assay in which substrate concentration is much lower than Km, the rate:

(a) Is independent of temperature
(b) Is independent of enzyme concentration
(c) Is proportional to substrate concentration
(d) Approaches Vmax.

58. The enzyme that catalyses the reaction $2\ H_2O \rightarrow 2\ H_2O + O_2$ is a:

(a) Dehydrogenase
(b) Peroxidase
(c) Catalase
(d) Hydrolase

59. The isocitrate dehydrogenase reaction is analogous to:

(a) Pyruvate dehydrogenase
(b) α-Ketoglutarate dehydrogenase
(c) Lactate dehydrogenase
(d) 6-phosphogluconate dehydrogenase

60. Dinitrophenol would be most likely to inhibit cell function by disrupting:

(a) TCA cycle
(b) Glycolysis
(c) Hepatic gluconeogenesis
(d) Oxidative phosphorylation

61. Protein that contain a porphyrin ring include:

(a) Catalase
(b) Cytochrome
(c) Hemoglobin
(d) All of them

62. Heavy chains of IgG antibody may be separated from the light chains with:

(a) Ethanolamine
(b) Pepsin
(c) Papain
(d) Mercaptoethanol

63. Isomerases are the enzymes that catalyze following changes within one molecule:

(a) Goemetric
(b) Structural
(c) Either of the two
(d) None of them

64. Km is:

(a) Dissociation constant for enzyme substrate complex:

(b) Equal to half the substrate concentration required to achieve Vmax

(c) The substrate concentration that give one half Vmax

(d) None of them

65. Isoenzymes are:

(a) Enzymes that exist in more than one amino acid sequence in same species

(b) Have identical catalytic properties

(c) Are single polypeptide chains that differ by an amino acid replacement

(d) None of them

66. Which of the following is an essential cofactor in carboxylation reactions:

(a) CoA (b) CTP

(c) Lipoic acid (d) Biotin

67. Which enzyme will cleave leucyl-glycyl-proline to leucine and glycyl proline?

(a) Carboxypeptidase (b) Chymotrypsin

(c) Aminopeptidase (d) Trypsin

68. Which of the following statements about isozymes of a given enzyme are true:

(a) They may exhibit different Km values for substrates

(b) Composed of different multimeric complexs

(c) Both (a) and (b)

(d) None of them

69. Which of the following proteins contain iron?

(a) Hemoglobin (b) Cytochrome C

(c) Myoglobin (d) All of them

70. The model for allosteric enzymes assume that:

(a) All are polymers

(b) Each sub unit bears catalytic and allosteric site

(c) Both (a) and (b)

(d) None of them

71. Phosphorylation sites in the mitochondrial respiratory chain may occur between:

(a) NAD and a flavoprotein

(b) Cytochrome b and cytochrome C

(c) Both (a) and (b)

(d) None of them

72. Which of the following statements about sickle cell anemia are true?

(a) Results from a single amino acid change in hemoglobin

(b) Seen in homozygous individual only

(c) Both (a) and (b)

(d) None of them

73. Most of the enzymes:

(a) Most active near neutral pH

(b) Increase the rapidity of reaction they catalyze

(c) Specific for substrate as well as the reaction catalyzed

(d) All of them

74. Which of the following statements concerning trypsinogen and chymotrypsinogen are false:

(a) Secreted by exocrine cells in the pancreas

(b) Have considerable homologies in primary sequence

(c) They are exopeptidases

(d) None of them

75. The isoenzymes of lactate dehydrogenase:

(a) Range from monomers to tetramers

(b) Differ only in single amino acid

(c) Exist in 5 forms depending upon the content M and H monomers

(d) None of them

76. The nerve gas, DFP has been useful reagent in enzyme chemistry. At the active site of many hydrolytic enzymes DFP combines with:

(a) Histidine
(b) Tryptophan

(c) Lysine
(d) Serine

77. Antimetabolites act by:

(a) Competitive inhibition when they combine irreversibly with an enzyme

(b) Competitive inhibition when they combine reversibly with an enzyme

(c) Non-competitive inhibition by combining with prosthetic group of enzyme

(d) None of them

78. Which of the statements about myosin is true?

(a) Low in α-helix content (b) Actin-binding protein

(c) Zinc requiring enzyme (d) None of them

79. Control of metabolic pathway may be exerted by enzyme repression. In vertebrates, this form of enzyme control occurs primarily in the;

(a) Heart (b) Brain

(c) Liver (d) Skeletal muscle

80. *De novo* **synthesis of enzyme, promoted by the substrate on which it acts, is characterized by the term:**

(a) Induction (b) Activation

(c) Derepression (d) None of them

81. Some antibiotics act as ionophores which mean that they:

(a) Inhibit both translation and transcription

(b) Inhibit only translation

(c) Increase cell membrane permeability to specific ions

(d) None of them

82. Which of the following oxidation reduction system has a highest redox potential:

(a) Fumarate/succinate (b) Fe^{+++} Cytochrome a/Fe^{++}

(c) NAD^+/NADH (d) None of them

83. Polymyxin is unique among chemotherapeutic agents, because it is bactericidal in absence of cell growth. It exerts it effect by:

(a) Binding to DNA polymerase

(b) Binding to polysome bound m-RNA

(c) Detergent like disruption of membranes

(d) None of them

84. Cycloserine inhibits transpeptidation in the formation of peptidoglycan cell wall network of gram-positive organisms. This action of cycloserine is competitively inhibited by:

(a) L-Lysine
(b) D-alanine
(c) D-glutamine
(d) D-serine

85. The example of transglycosidase:

(a) Hexokinase
(b) Phosphorylase
(c) GPT
(d) None of them

86. Pepsin works only in:

(a) Acid medium
(b) Alkaline medium
(c) Neutral medium
(d) None of them

87. At 0°C, most of the enzymes are:

(a) Active
(b) Inactive
(c) Neutral
(d) None of them

88. The substrate concentration that produces half maximal velocity is known as:

(a) Michaelis constant
(b) Km value,
(c) Either of the two
(d) Neither of the two

89. With enzymes many substrates form:

(a) 1 bond
(b) 2 bonds
(c) 3 bonds
(d) None of them

90. Many enzymes are:

(a) Conjugated protein
(b) Derived protein
(c) Simple protein
(d) None of them

91. Lysozome has a central catalytic site with subunits:

(a) 4
(b) 5
(c) 6
(d) 8

92. Potassium containing enzyme is:

(a) Pyruvate Kinase
(b) Urease
(c) Xanthine oxidase
(d) None of them

93. Nickel containing enzyme is:

(a) Urease
(b) Xanthine oxidase
(c) Pyruvate kinase
(d) All of them

94. Serum trypsin level is increased in:

(a) Diseases of pancreas (b) Diseases of liver

(c) Diseases of kidney (d) None of them

95. Serum lipase level is decreased in:

(a) Vitamin A deficiency (b) Diabetes mellitus

(c) Both (a) and (b) (d) None of them

96. Serum cholinesterase level is increased in:

(a) Nephrotic syndrome (b) Muscle trauma

(c) Viral hepatitis (d) None of them

97. AST is higher than ALT in:

(a) Cirrhosis (b) Hemolytic jaundice

(c) Both (a) and (b) (d) None of them

98. CPK is apparently not present in:

(a) Liver (b) Kidney

(c) Erythrocytes (d) All of them

99. Serum isocitrate dehydrogenase level is increased in:

(a) Kidney diseases (b) Liver diseases

(c) Pancreatic diseases (d) None of them

100. Serum amylase concentration is decreased in:

(a) Pancreatic diseases (b) Liver diseases

(c) Kidney diseases (d) None of them

Answer Key

1	(d)	26	(c)	51	(d)	76	(d)
2	(a)	27	(a)	52	(d)	77	(b)
3	(b)	28	(c)	53	(a)	78	(b)
4	(d)	29	(b)	54	(b)	79	(c)
5	(c)	30	(a)	55	(a)	80	(a)
6	(d)	31	(a)	56	(d)	81	(c)
7	(a)	32	(c)	57	(c)	82	(b)
8	(d)	33	(b)	58	(c)	83	(c)
9	(c)	34	(d)	59	(d)	84	(b)
10	(a)	35	(c)	60	(d)	85	(b)
11	(c)	36	(d)	61	(d)	86	(a)
12	(a)	37	(a)	62	(d)	87	(b)
13	(a)	38	(b)	63	(c)	88	(c)
14	(b)	39	(b)	64	(c)	89	(c)
15	(c)	40	(c)	65	(d)	90	(c)
16	(c)	41	(c)	66	(d)	91	(c)
17	(a)	42	(d)	67	(c)	92	(a)
18	(c)	43	(c)	68	(c)	93	(a)
19	(c)	44	(c)	69	(d)	94	(a)
20	(c)	45	(a)	70	(c)	95	(c)
21	(c)	46	(a)	71	(c)	96	(a)
22	(c)	47	(a)	72	(c)	97	(c)
23	(a)	48	(d)	73	(d)	98	(d)
24	(c)	49	(b)	74	(c)	99	(b)
25	(a)	50	(d)	75	(c)	100	(b)

Chapter 8

Vitamins

1. **The metabolite excreted in urine in thiamine deficiency:**
   (a) Pyruvate (b) Glucose
   (c) Xanthurenic acid (d) FIGLU
2. **The coenzyme directly concerned with the synthesis of biogenic amines:**
   (a) TPP (b) $NADP^+$
   (c) Biotin (d) Pyridoxal phosphate
3. **Folic acid antagonist used in the treatment of cancer:**
   (a) Methotrexate (b) Trimethoprim
   (c) Sulfonamide (d) All the three
4. **The three Ds in pellagra stands for:**
   (a) Dermatitis (b) Dementia
   (c) Diarrhoea (d) All the three
5. **Which of the following 2 pairs resemble in their function:**
   (a) Carbohydrates and proteins (b) Proteins and lipids
   (c) Proteins and hormones (d) Vitamins and hormones
6. **Pick up the fat insoluble vitamin:**
   (a) A (b) C
   (c) D (d) E

7. Which of the following is incorrect about fat soluble vitamin:

(a) Soluble in fat

(b) Require bile salt for absorption

(c) Not stored in the body

(d) Normally not excreted in urine

8. The most important pro vitamin A is:

(a) α-carotene (b) β-carotene

(c) γ-carotene (d) All of them

9. Retinol exists mainly as an ester with palmitic acid in:

(a) Liver (b) Lung

(c) Fat depots (d) All the three

10. Which is the most important organ regarding the storage of vitamin A?

(a) Liver (b) Lung

(c) Kidney (d) Fat depots

11. Retinol is distributed to various organs in the form of protein complex having:

(a) α_1-globulin (b) α_2-globulin

(c) β-globulin (d) γ-globulin

12. Carotenes are transported with the:

(a) Protein (b) Lipids

(c) Lipoproteins (d) Minerals

13. The I.U. is equal to the number of micrograms of β-carotene:

(a) 0.3 (b) 0.4

(c) 0.6 (d) 0.8

14. Under normal conditions very small amount of vitamin A is excreted through:

(a) Urine (b) Feces

(c) Sweat (d) All the three

15. Color blindness is due to the deficiency of:

(a) Cone and rod pigments (b) Cone pigments

(c) Rod pigments (d) None of them

16. The rod and cone pigments are protein complexes. The non-prosthetic group of these complexes is:

(a) Only retinal (b) Only retinol

(c) Retinal and retinol (d) Retinol and dehydroretinol

17. The preformed vitamin A is supplied by foods such as:

(a) Eggs (b) Butter

(c) Fish liver (d) All of them

18. In the night blindness, patient is unable to resynthesize:

(a) Retinal (b) Retinol

(c) Retinene (d) Rhodopsin

19. Vitamin A is a specific treatment for the cure and prevention of:

(a) Xeropthalmia (b) Nyctalopia

(c) Hemeralopia (d) All the three

20. Continued intake of excessive amount of vitamin A especially in children produces:

(a) Irritability (b) Anorexia

(c) Headache (d) All of them

21. Hypervitaminosis of retinol is mainly due to:

(a) Occurence in bulk in usual diet (b) Its degradation

(c) Difficulty in transportation (d) Difficulty in excretion

22. Viosterol is an alternate name of:

(a) Vitamin A_1 (b) Vitamin A_2

(c) Vitamin D_2 (d) Vitamin D_3

23. Exposure of skin to sunlight leads to the production of cholecalciferol the precursor of which is:

(a) Cholesterol (b) 7-dehydrocholesterol

(c) Ergosterol (d) Ergocalciferol

24. Which of the following is quite stable to heat:

(a) Vitamin D_2 (b) Vitamin D_3

(c) Both (a) and (b) (d) None of them

25. Milk is the poor source of:

(a) Vitamin A (b) Vitamin B_2

(c) Vitamin D (d) None of them

26. Tocopherols prevent the oxidation of:

(a) Vitamin A (b) Vitamin C

(c) Vitamin D (d) Vitamin K

27. Which of the tocopherols is the most potent antioxidant:

(a) α (b) β

(c) γ (d) δ

28. The activity of tocopherols is destroyed by:

(a) Oxidation (b) Reduction

(c) Conjugation (d) All of them

29. Vitamin E is stored in:

(a) Mitochondria (b) Microsomes

(c) Both (a) and (b) (d) None of them

30. Vitamin K_2 also known as farnoquinone is found in:

(a) Alfalfa (b) Carrot tops

(c) Cabbage (d) Bacteria

31. The principal overall effect of vitamin K is to shorten the prothrombin time to:

(a) 0-5 Sec. (b) 12-15 Sec.

(c) 15-20 Sec. (d) 20-25 Sec.

32. The deficiency of vitamin K can be removed by:

(a) 1,4 naphthaquinone (b) Menadione

(c) Phthiocol (d) All of them

33. The co-enzyme co-carboxylase has a vitamin in its structure which is:

(a) Vitamin B_1 (b) Vitamin B_2

(c) Vitamin B_6 (d) Vitamin A_1

34. Which is not a good source of thiamine?

(a) Pulses (b) Nuts

(c) White flour (d) Whole meal flour

35. The most important store house of vitamin B_1 is:

(a) Liver (b) Heart

(c) Brain (d) Kidney

36. The requirement of vitamin B_1 is increased in case of:

(a) Fever (b) Increased muscular activity

(c) Hyperthyroidism (d) All of them

37. Riboflavin molecule contains:

(a) D-ribose (b) D-ribitol

(c) D-2-deoxyribose (d) D-2-deoxyribitol

38. Which of the following vitamin A functions as a steroid hormone:

(a) Retinal (b) Retinol

(c) Retinoic acid (d) β-carotene

39. Major form of vitamin D in circulation is:

(a) Cholecalciferol (b) 25-hydroxycholecalciferol

(c) 24,25 dihydroxycholecalciferol (d) None of them

40. The most important source of riboflavin is:

(a) Liver (b) Yeast

(c) Egg (d) Milk

41. The normal concentration of riboflavin per 100ml plasma is:

(a) 1.5-3.5mg (b) 2.5-4.0mg

(c) 3.5-5.5mg (d) 4.5-7.5mg

42. Riboflavin is involved in the regulatory function of some hormones connected with the metabolism of:

(a) Carbohydrates (b) Fats

(c) Proteins (d) Minerals

43. Deficiency of riboflavin causes:

(a) Cheilosis (b) Glossitis

(c) Angular somatitis (d) All of them

44. In the oxidation reaction catalyzed by riboflavin enzymes, reaction occurs at which part of the enzyme?

(a) Ribose (b) Flavin

(c) Adenine (d) Either of the three

45. DDD (Three D's) are the symptoms associated with the deficiency of vitamin:

(a) D (b) B_1

(c) B_2 (d) B_5

46. Niacin is:

(a) Pyridine-1-carboxylic acid
(b) Pyridine-2-carboxylic acid
(c) Pyridine-3-carboxylic acid
(d) Pyridine-4-carboxylic acid

47. The best source of nicotinamide is:

(a) Bran
(b) Egg
(c) Milk
(d) Fruits

48. In maize niacin is present in the form of:

(a) Niacin
(b) Nicotine
(c) Niacytin
(d) Nicyn

49. The deficiency of nicotinic acid may overcome by administering:

(a) Glycine
(b) Alanine
(c) Tyrosine
(d) Tryptophan

50. Majority of the nicotinic acid excreted in urine is in the form of:

(a) Free nicotinic acid
(b) N-methyl nicotinic acid
(c) Both (a) and (b)
(d) None of them

51. Nicotinic acid is essential for the functioning of:

(a) Skin
(b) Digestive system
(c) Nervous system
(d) All of them

52. Pyridoxal phosphate is involved in which of the following reaction of α-amino acid?

(a) Transamination
(b) Decarboxylation
(c) Elimination
(d) All of them

53. Which of the following is pyridoxine antagonist?

(a) Deoxypyridoxine
(b) Isoniazid
(c) Both (a) and (b)
(d) Neither of the two

54. Pentathenic acid exists in the tissues as:

(a) β-mercaptoethylamine
(b) Co-enzyme A
(c) Pentoic acid
(d) β-alanine

55. Which amino acid is present in folic acid?

(a) Tryptophan
(b) Tyrosine
(c) Glutamine
(d) Glutamic acid

56. Which of the vitamin is involved in the metabolism of one-carbon fragment?

(a) B_1
(b) B_2
(c) B_9
(d) B_6

57. The vitamin involved in the formation of red blood cells is:

(a) B_2
(b) B_9
(c) B_6
(d) B_{12}

58. Vitamin C is:

(a) D-ascorbic acid
(b) L-ascorbic acid
(c) Either of the two
(d) Neither of the two

59. Ascorbic acid is destroyed in presence of:

(a) Light
(b) Oxygen
(c) Heat
(d) All of them

60. Deficiency symptoms of vitamin C are:

(a) Swollen bleeding gums
(b) Poor healing wounds
(c) Loss of appetite and weight
(d) All of them

61. The vitamin required on micro scale by human is:

(a) A
(b) B-complex
(c) C
(d) D

62. As an antioxidant, vitamin C reduces the risk of:

(a) Cancer
(b) Cataract
(c) Coronary heart disease
(d) All of them

63. Antagonist to vitamin K is:

(a) Heparin
(b) Bis-hydroxy coumarin
(c) Both (a) and (b)
(d) None of them

64. Administration of large doses of vitamin K produces:

(a) Hemolytic anemia
(b) Jaundice
(c) Both (a) and (b)
(d) None of them

65. Vitamin K's activity is lost by:

(a) Oxidizing agents
(b) Strong acids
(c) Irradiation
(d) All of them

66. Vitamin E is:

(a) Antioxidant
(b) Anti sterile
(c) Both (a) and (b)
(d) None of them

67. Deficiency symptoms of vitamin E are:

(a) Megaloblastic anemia
(b) Degenerative changes in muscles
(c) Changes in central nervous system
(d) All of them

68. High consumption of vitamin D is associated with:

(a) Loss of appetite
(b) Nausea
(c) Loss of weight
(d) All of them

69. Excess consumption of vitamin A leads to:

(a) Dermatitis
(b) Enlargement of liver
(c) Weight Loss
(d) All of them

70. Retinal is reduced to retinol by retinene reductase in presence of co-enzyme:

(a) NAD^+
(b) $NADP^+$
(c) NADH+ H+
(d) $NADPH + H^+$

71. The dietary vitamin A which is the form of vitamin A esters are hydrolyzed in the lumen of intestine by the enzyme:

(a) Amylase
(b) Lipase
(c) Peptidase
(d) Nuclease

72. In the blood vitamin esters are attached to:

(a) α_1-lipoproteins
(b) α_2-lipoproteins
(c) β-lipoproteins
(d) γ-lipoproteins

73. The percentage of vitamin A in the ester form is stored in the liver is:

(a) 80
(b) 85
(c) 90
(d) 95

74. The non-protein part of rhodopsin is:

(a) Retinal
(b) Retinol
(c) Carotene
(d) Repsin

75. Lumirhodopsin is stable only at a temperature below:

(a) -35°C (b) -40°C
(c) -45°C (d) -50°C

76. The normal concentration of vitamin A in blood in IU/dl:

(a) 20-25 (b) 24-60
(c) 30-65 (d) 35-70

77. Vitamin D_2 is also said to be:

(a) Activated ergosterol (b) Ergocalciferol
(c) Viosterol (d) All of them

78. Metarhodopsin is hydrolyzed to retinal and opsin at a temperature below:

(a) -8°C (b) -10°C
(c) -15°C (d) -20°C

79. The poor source of vitamin D:

(a) Egg (b) Butter
(c) Milk (d) Liver

80. The normal concentration of Vitamin D in blood in IU/L:

(a) 600-2500 (b) 700-3100
(c) 800-4100 (d) 850-4700

81. Some tocopherols are:

(a) Terpenoid in structure (b) Dionol in structure
(c) Isoprenoid in structure (d) Farnesyl in strcutre

82. The methyl groups in the aromatic nucleus of α-tocopherol are:

(a) 2 (b) 3
(c) 4 (d) 5

83. Vitamin E protects the polyunsaturated fatty acids from oxidation by molecular oxygen in the formation of:

(a) Superoxide (b) Peroxide
(c) Trioxide (d) All of them

84. Vitamin E protects enzymes from destruction in:

(a) Muscles (b) Nerves
(c) Gonads (d) All of them

85. The poor sources of vitamin K_1 are:

(a) Milk
(b) Meat
(c) Fish
(d) All of them

86. Vitamin K regulates the synthesis of blood clotting factors:

(a) VII
(b) IX
(c) X
(d) All of them

87. Ascorbic acid can reduce:

(a) 2,6- dichlorophenol indophenol
(b) 2,4- dinitrobenzene
(c) 2,6- dioxypyridine
(d) 2,6- dibromobenzene

88. Vitamin C is required in the metabolism of:

(a) Phenylalanine
(b) Tryptophan
(c) Both (a) and (b)
(d) None of them

89. The symptoms of scurvy are:

(a) Poor healing of wounds
(b) Loosening of teeth
(c) Anemia
(d) All of them

90. Thiamine is also said to be:

(a) Anti beri beri substance
(b) Antineuritic Vitamin
(c) Aneurine
(d) All of them

91. Lipoic acid is also termed as:

(a) Thioctic acid
(b) Protogen
(c) Acetate replacement factor
(d) All of them

92. Folic acid is also termed as:

(a) SLR factor
(b) Pteroyl-glutamic acid
(c) Liver lactobacillus casei factor
(d) Both (b) and (c)

93. Thiamine is oxidized to thiochrome in alkaline solution by:

(a) Potassium permanganate
(b) Potassium ferricyanide
(c) Potassium dichromate
(d) Potassium chlorate

94. Riboflavin in alkaline solution when exposed to ultraviolet light is converted into lumiflavin which in ultraviolet light has a:

(a) Greenish yellow fluorescence
(b) Bluish yellow fluorescence
(c) Reddish yellow fluorescence
(d) Light yellow fluorescence

95. FMN is a constituent of the:

(a) Warburg yellow enzyme
(b) Cytochrome C reductase
(c) L-amino acid dehydrogenase
(d) All of them

96. The majority of the excess of nicotinic acid is excreted in the urine in the form of:

(a) N-methyl nicotinamide
(b) 6-pyridone of N-methyl nicotinamide
(c) N-methyl nicotinic acid
(d) All of them

97. The normal concentration of niacin in blood in mg/100ml:

(a) 0.3 to 0.5
(b) 0.4 to 0.6
(c) 0.5 to 0.8
(d) 0.6 to 0.9

98. Nicotinic acid is essential for the functioning of:

(a) Skin
(b) intestinal tract
(c) Nervous system
(d) All of them

99. Pyridoxine is a mixture of:

(a) Pyridoxine
(b) Pyridoxal
(c) Pyridoxamine
(d) All of them

100. Pyridoxine produces a coloured compound with:

(a) 2,6- dichloroquinone chlorimide
(b) 2,6-dichloroquinone
(c) 2,4- nitroquinone
(d) All of them

101. Pyridoxine phosphate is involved in the desulphuration of:

(a) Cysteine
(b) Homocysteine
(c) Both (a) and (b)
(d) None of them

102. In some subjects pyridoxine deficiency causes:

(a) Lymphopenia
(b) Peripheral neuropathy
(c) Both (a) and (b)
(d) None of them

103. In the deficiency states of vitamin B_6, there are inborn errors of metabolism including:

(a) Cystathioninuria
(b) Fimilial xanthurenic aciduria
(c) Anemias
(d) All of them

104. Pentothenic acid deficiency causes:

(a) Nausea (b) Irritability
(c) Anemia (d) All of them

105. Folic acid co-enzymes take part in the synthesis of:

(a) Purines (b) Thymine
(c) Both (a) and (b) (d) None of them

106. Folic acid inhibitors are:

(a) Aminopterine (b) Amethopterine
(c) Both (a) and (b) (d) None of them

107. Vitamin B_{12} binds to the proteins of:

(a) Gastric juice (b) Bile
(c) Saliva (d) All of them

108. Osteomalacia can be prevented by the administration of:

(a) Vitamin D (b) Calcium
(c) Both (a) and (b) (d) None of them

109. In pernicious anemia, the tongue is:

(a) Sored (b) Inflammated
(c) Both (a) and (b) (d) None of them

110. The antagonists of vitamin B_6 are:

(a) Isonicotinic acid hydrazide (b) Hydralazine
(c) Both (a) and (b) (d) None of them

111. The phospholipids of mitochondria possess affinities for:

(a) α-tocopherol (b) Vitamin E
(c) Both (a) and (b) (d) None of them

112. Flavoproteins form metalloflavoproteins by uniting with metals like:

(a) Iron (b) Molybdenum
(c) Both (a) and (b) (d) None of them

113. Fat soluble vitamins include:

(a) Folic acid (b) Vitamin K
(c) Riboflavin (d) Ascorbic acid

114. Vitamin C is:

(a) Strongly acid (b) Mild acid
(c) A base (d) None of them

115. The Disease resulting from vitamin C deficiency is:

(a) Pernicious anemia (b) Beri beri
(c) Keratomalacia (d) None of them

116. Ascorbic acid deficiency affects the formation of:

(a) Collagen (b) Myosin
(c) Keratin (d) Histone

117. 7-dehydrocholesterol is found in:

(a) Skin (b) Sebum
(c) Both (a) and (b) (d) None of them

118. Absence of vitamin D causes:

(a) Osteomalacia (b) Myocardial infarction
(c) Dermatosis (d) None of them

119. 7-dehydrochloesterol gets changed into vitamin D in presence of:

(a) Ultraviolet light (b) Dim light
(c) Infrared light (d) None of them

120. Epimers of tocopherol include:

(a) α (b) β
(c) γ (d) All of them

121. Vitamin K_2 has a different side chain which is known as:

(a) Farnesyl (b) Phytyl
(c) Both (a) and (b) (d) None of them

122. The most serious deficiency disease of vitamin B_1 is:

(a) Rickets (b) Sterility
(c) Beri-beri (d) Pellagra

123. Vitamin thiamine is also known as:

(a) B_1 (b) Aneurin
(c) Both (a) and (b) (d) None of them

124. Keratomalacia means:

(a) Irreversible corneal opacity (b) Irreversible dermatitis
(c) Irreversible conjuctivitis (d) Irreversible night blindness

125. Vitamin A deficiency in human beings causes:

(a) Xanthomatosis (b) Sterility
(c) Mental retardation (d) Keratomalacia

126. In human body some quantity of niacin is synthesized from:

(a) Tryptophan
(b) Tyrosine
(c) Phenylalanine
(d) Threonine

127. Pellagra disease is characterized by:

(a) Gastro enteritis
(b) Osteomalacia
(c) Exfoliative dermatitis
(d) Aplastic anemia

128. The flavin which is found in milk is known as:

(a) Lactoflavin
(b) Ovoflavin
(c) Hepatoflavin
(d) None of them

129. The flavin which is found in eggs is known as:

(a) Lactoflavin
(b) Ovoflavin
(c) Hepatoflavin
(d) None of them

130. Beri-beri is characterized by:

(a) Bradycardia
(b) Anorexia
(c) Both (a) and (b)
(d) None of them

131. Another name of folic acid is:

(a) Pteroylglutamic acid
(b) Glycinamide
(c) Pseudouridine
(d) None of them

132. Vitamin B_{12} plays a role in the formation and synthesis of:

(a) Carbohydrates
(b) Lipids
(c) Proteins
(d) Nucleic acids

133. Vitamin B_{12} increases the biosynthesis of methyl groups from precursors such as:

(a) α-Carbon of glycine
(b) β-carbon of glycine
(c) Both (a) and (b)
(d) None of them

134. Which metal is responsible for imparting deep red colour to vitamin B_{12}:

(a) Magnesium
(b) Manganese
(c) Cobalt
(d) Chromium

135. In pernicious anemia, the stomach loses, in middle life, the capacity to produce:

(a) An intrinsic factor
(b) An extrinsic factor
(c) Both (a) and (b)
(d) None of them

136. In the structure of Vitamin B_{12}, centrally placed cobalt remains attached to:

(a) Magnesium (b) Manganese

(c) Cyanide (d) Chloride

137. Choline as such is stored in the:

(a) Liver (b) Kidney

(c) Seeds (d) None of them

138. p-aminobenzoic acid is the bridge between pteroic acid and glutamic acid in the structure of:

(a) Vitamin B_{12} (b) Folic acid

(c) Pentothenic acid (d) Riboflavin

139. Which vitamin absorbs ultraviolet radiation (maximum 297.5mμ) in the range which produces sun burn and suntan in human skin:

(a) B_1 (b) B_2

(c) B_{12} (d) Para aminobenzoic acid

140. The co-enzyme form of niacin is also known as:

(a) NAD^+ (b) $NADP^+$

(c) DPN^+ (d) All of them

141. Lipoic acid in good amount is found in:

(a) Liver (b) Soybean meal

(c) Both (a) and (b) (d) None of them

142. The concentration of p-aminobenzoic acid in milk is about:

(a) 0.1mg/L (b) 0.5mg/L

(c) 1.0mg/L (d) 2.0mg/L

143. Characteristic signs of the deficiency of vitamin B_2 are:

(a) Cheilosis (b) Glossitis

(c) Both (a) and (b) (d) None of them

144. Xanthine oxidase contains the metal:

(a) Iron (b) Molybdenum

(c) Both (a) and (b) (d) None of them

145. Niacin is required for the synthesis of oxidative co-enzyme:

(a) NAD (b) NADP

(c) Both (a) and (b) (d) None of them

146. In man deficiency diseases of vitamin A are almost limited to the organ:

(a) Eyes (b) Ears

(c) Stomach (d) Intestine

147. Role of biotin as a key component in:

(a) Carboxylation (b) Decarboxylation

(c) Both (a) and (b) (d) None of them

148. Vitamin B_{12} is found in abundance in:

(a) Liver (b) Kidney

(c) Both (a) and (b) (d) None of them

149. The deficiency of choline in animals can be prevented by:

(a) Methionine (b) Betaine

(c) Both (a) and (b) (d) None of them

150. The best source of vitamin D is:

(a) Margarine (b) Vegetables

(c) Wheat (d) None of them

Answer Key

1	(a)	26	(a)	51	(d)	76	(b)
2	(d)	27	(d)	52	(d)	77	(d)
3	(a)	28	(a)	53	(c)	78	(c)
4	(d)	29	(c)	54	(b)	79	(c)
5	(d)	30	(d)	55	(d)	80	(b)
6	(b)	31	(b)	56	(c)	81	(a)
7	(c)	32	(d)	57	(d)	82	(b)
8	(b)	33	(a)	58	(b)	83	(b)
9	(d)	34	(c)	59	(d)	84	(d)
10	(a)	35	(b)	60	(d)	85	(d)
11	(a)	36	(d)	61	(c)	86	(d)
12	(c)	37	(b)	62	(d)	87	(a)
13	(c)	38	(b)	63	(c)	88	(c)
14	(b)	39	(b)	64	(c)	89	(d)
15	(b)	40	(b)	65	(d)	90	(d)
16	(d)	41	(b)	66	(c)	91	(d)
17	(d)	42	(a)	67	(d)	92	(d)
18	(d)	43	(d)	68	(d)	93	(b)
19	(d)	44	(b)	69	(d)	94	(a)
20	(d)	45	(d)	70	(c)	95	(d)
21	(d)	46	(c)	71	(b)	96	(d)
22	(c)	47	(a)	72	(c)	97	(c)
23	(b)	48	(c)	73	(d)	98	(d)
24	(c)	49	(d)	74	(a)	99	(d)
25	(c)	50	(b)	75	(d)	100	(a)

101	**(c)**	**114**	**(a)**	**127**	**(c)**	**140**	**(d)**
102	**(c)**	**115**	**(d)**	**128**	**(a)**	**141**	**(c)**
103	**(d)**	**116**	**(a)**	**129**	**(b)**	**142**	**(a)**
104	**(d)**	**117**	**(c)**	**130**	**(c)**	**143**	**(c)**
105	**(c)**	**118**	**(a)**	**131**	**(a)**	**144**	**(c)**
106	**(c)**	**119**	**(a)**	**132**	**(d)**	**145**	**(c)**
107	**(d)**	**120**	**(d)**	**133**	**(c)**	**146**	**(a)**
108	**(c)**	**121**	**(a)**	**134**	**(c)**	**147**	**(c)**
109	**(c)**	**122**	**(c)**	**135**	**(c)**	**148**	**(d)**
110	**(c)**	**123**	**(c)**	**136**	**(c)**	**149**	**(c)**
111	**(c)**	**124**	**(a)**	**137**	**(d)**	**150**	**(a)**
112	**(c)**	**125**	**(d)**	**138**	**(b)**		
113	**(b)**	**126**	**(a)**	**139**	**(d)**		

Chapter 9

Hormones

1. **Insulin has the influence on the metabolism of:**
   (a) Carbohydrates (b) Proteins
   (c) Fats (d) All of them

2. **During fasting hormonal changes occur that promote:**
   (a) Glycogenesis (b) Lipogenesis
   (c) Lipolysis (d) Glycolysis

3. **From bones in animals parathormone hormone mobilize:**
   (a) Calcium (b) Phosphorus
   (c) Both (a) and (b) (d) None of them

4. **Proliferation of vaginal epithelium and endometrium is observed after the administration of:**
   (a) Oestrogen (b) Progesterone
   (c) Both (a) and (b) (d) None of them

5. **Contraction of smooth muscles is the function of:**
   (a) Oxytocin (b) Vasopressin
   (c) Both (a) and (b) (d) None of them

6. **Presence of glucose in blood inhibits the secretion of:**
   (a) Insulin (b) Glucagon
   (c) Both (a) and (b) (d) None of them

7. **Na^+ reabsorption by renal tubules is increased by the hormone:**
   (a) Aldosterone
   (b) Testosterone
   (c) Both (a) and (b)
   (d) None of them

8. **The endocrine organ responsible for synthesis of trophic hormone:**
   (a) Anterior pituitary
   (b) Posterior pituitary
   (c) Both (a) and (b)
   (d) None of them

9. **Substrate cycling is stimulated by:**
   (a) Growth hormone
   (b) Thyroid hormone
   (c) Both (a) and (b)
   (d) None of them

10. **Calves fed a milk diet that may lead to hypomagnesia develop a decreased activity of:**
    (a) Thyroid
    (b) Insulin
    (c) Glucagon
    (d) Epinephrine

11. **Diabetes mellitus caused by the deficiency of the secretion of:**
    (a) Insulin
    (b) Glucagon
    (c) Both (a) and (b)
    (d) None of them

12. **cAMP is formed from ATP by enzyme adenyl cyclase which is activated by the hormone:**
    (a) Insulin
    (b) Epinephrine
    (c) Testosterone
    (d) Progesterone

13. **In most cases the circulating hormone levels are regulated by:**
    (a) Negative feedback
    (b) Positive feedback
    (c) Both (a) and (b)
    (d) None of them

14. **Glycogenolysis in liver is stimulated by:**
    (a) Epinephrine
    (b) Cortisol
    (c) GH
    (d) Aldosterone

15. **One of the following hormones is an amino acid derivative:**
    (a) Epinephrine
    (b) Nor-epinephrine
    (c) Thyroxine
    (d) All of them

16. **The most active mineralocorticoid hormone is:**
    (a) Cortisol
    (b) Aldosterone
    (c) II-Deoxy corticosterone
    (d) Corticosterone

17. BMR test is done to assess the activity of:

(a) Adrenaline (b) Oestrogen

(c) Thyroxine (d) Insulin

18. Epinephrine is formed from nor-epinephrine by:

(a) N-Methylation (b) Decarboxylation

(c) Hydroxylation (d) Transamination

19. Which of the following hormones is involved in increased reabsorption of water from renal epithelial cells:

(a) Insulin (b) Vasopressin

(c) Epinephrine (d) Cortisol

20. The most potent mineralocorticoid is:

(a) Aldosterone (b) Cortisol

(c) Corticosterone (d) None of them

21. The hormone regulating the calcium homeostasis include:

(a) Parathormone (b) Calcitonin

(c) Vitamin D (d) All of them

22. The transport of glucose across the cell membrane is facilitated by:

(a) Glucagon (b) Insulin

(c) Thyroxine (d) Gonadotrophin

23. Which of the following has important role in maintenance of ECV:

(a) ADH (b) Rennin-Angiotensin

(c) Cortisol (d) None of them

24. Molecular weight of parathormone is:

(a) 8500 (b) 9000

(c) 10000 (d) 20000

25. The hormone that stimulates the release of bile from gall bladder is:

(a) Insulin (b) Secretin

(c) Hepatocrinin (d) Cholecystokinin

26. The hormones that differ least in chemical structure are:

(a) Insulin and Proinsulin

(b) Oxytocin and Vasopressin

(c) Cortisone and growth stimulating hormone

(d) Thyrotropin and oxytocin

27. Name of hormone predominantly produced in flight, fright and fight:

(a) Thyroxine (b) Aldosterone

(c) Epinephrine (d) ADH

28. The hormone essentially required for the implantation of fertilized ovum and maintenance of pregnancy:

(a) Progesterone (b) Oestrogen

(c) Cortisol (d) Prolactin

29. The inorganic ion that can act as a second messenger for certain hormones is:

(a) Ca^{2+} (b) Na^{+}

(c) K^{+} (d) None of them

30. The compounds that produce opiate like effects on the central nervous system are:

(a) Endorphins (b) Enkephalins

(c) Both (a) and (b) (d) None of them

31. Impairment in the synthesis of dopamine by the brain is a causative factor for the disorder:

(a) Parkinson's disease (b) Addison's disease

(c) Cushing syndrome (d) Goitre

32. Hormones are produced by endocrine glands to control:

(a) Metabolic activity (b) Biological activity

(c) Both (a) and (b) (d) None of them

33. Group I hormones are derivatives of cholesterol except:

(a) T_3 (b) T_4

(c) Both (a) and (b) (d) None of them

34. Hormones (Group I) act through intracellular receptors located in:

(a) Cytoplasm (b) Nucleus

(c) Either (a) or (b) (d) Neither (a) or (b)

35. The hormonal action mediated through intracellular receptors is not immediate since sufficient time is needed for:

(a) Transcription (b) Translation

(c) Both (a) and (b) (d) None of them

36. Hormone action is regulated by:
(a) Rate of synthesis and secretion
(b) Specific transport system in plasma
(c) Hormone specific receptors in target cell membrane
(d) All of them

37. Group II hormones are:
(a) Hydrophilic (b) Lyophilic
(c) Hydrophobic (d) None of them

38. The action of most protein hormones is inhibited:
(a) In presence of calcium (b) In absence of calcium
(c) Either of the two (d) Neither of the two

39. Somatotropin has amino acids:
(a) 191 (b) 189
(c) 187 (d) None of them

40. Somatotropin increases the synthesis of:
(a) DNA (b) RNA
(c) Collagen (d) All of them

41. Somatotropin promotes the retention of:
(a) Calcium (b) Phosphorus
(c) Both (a) and (b) (d) None of them

42. Prolactin stimulates:
(a) Mammary growth (b) Milk secretion
(c) mRNA synthesis (d) All of them

43. Thyroid stimulating hormone stimulates:
(a) Phospholipid synthesis (b) TCA cycle
(c) Glycolysis (d) All of them

44. Adrenocorticotropic hormone has amino acids in number:
(a) 39 (b) 29
(c) 35 (d) None of them

45. Molecular weight of follicle stimulating hormone:
(a) 25000 (b) 40000
(c) Either (a) or (b) (d) Neither (a) or (b)

46. Oxytocin differs from vasopressin with respect to:

(a) 3rd and 8th amino acid residues

(b) 2nd and 7th amino acid residues

(c) 1st and 6th amino acid residues

(d) None of them

47. Thyroid hormones increase hepatic:

(a) Gluconeogenesis (b) Glycogenolysis

(c) Both (a) and (b) (d) None of them

48. Thyroid hormones increase:

(a) Lipolysis (b) Plasma lipoprotein

(c) Both (a) and (b) (d) None of them

49. Parathormone increases:

(a) Serum Ca^{++} (b) Urinary Ca^{++}

(c) Urinary PO_4 (d) All of them

50. Parathormone inhibits trans-membrane transport of:

(a) K^+ (b) HCO^-_3

(c) Both (a) and (b) (d) None of them

51. Calcitonin decreases the activity of:

(a) Lysosomal hydrolases (b) Pyrophosphatase

(c) Alkaline phosphatase in bones (d) All of them

52. Major target tissues of insulin are:

(a) Muscle (b) Liver

(c) Adipose tissue (d) All of them

53. Insulin is inactivated by:

(a) Breaking of disulphide bond

(b) Digestion with proteolytic enzymes

(c) Both (a) and (b)

(d) None of them

54. Insulin increases:

(a) Glycolysis (b) Glycogenesis

(c) HMP Shunt (d) All of them

55. Insulin decreases:

(a) Lipolysis (b) Ketogenesis

(c) Both (a) and (b) (d) None of them

56. Insulin decreases:

(a) K^+ concentration in blood (b) Inorganic P in blood

(c) Both (a) and (b) (d) None of them

57. Glucagon increases:

(a) Protein catabolism (b) Urinary NPN

(c) Urea (d) All of them

58. Glucagon increases:

(a) Release of calcitonin from thyroid (b) K^+ release from liver

(c) Both (a) and (b) (d) None of them

59. Somatostatin inhibits the secretion of:

(a) Insulin (b) Glucagon

(c) Both (a) and (b) (d) None of them

60. Epinephrine inhibits the secretion of:

(a) Insulin (b) Glucagon

(c) Somatotropin (d) None of them

61. Epinephrine and norepinephrine increase:

(a) Glycogenolysis (b) Gluconeogenesis

(c) Both (a) and (b) (d) None of them

62. Parkinson's disease is characterized by:

(a) Muscular rigidity (b) Tremors

(c) Involuntary movements (d) All of them

63. Iodide transport is inhibited by antithyroid agents like:

(a) Thiocyanate (b) Perchlorate

(c) Both (a) and (b) (d) None of them

64. In its biological functions T_3 is active then T_4:

(a) 4 times (b) 3 times

(c) 2 times (d) None of them

65. Thyroid hormones increase the oxygen consumption in most of the tissue except:

(a) Brain (b) Lungs
(c) Testes (d) All of them

66. Thyroid hormones cause positive nitrogen balance and promote:

(a) Growth (b) Development
(c) Both (a) and (b) (d) None of them

67. Thyroid hormones regulate the metabolism of:

(a) Water (b) Electrolyte
(c) Both (a) and (b) (d) None of them

68. The drugs which interfere with the production of thyroid hormones are:

(a) Thiourea (b) Thiouracil
(c) Thiocarbamid (d)All of them

69. Hyperthyroidism is characterized by :

(a) Increased metabolic rate (b) Nervousness
(c) Rapid heart rate (d) All of them

70. Hyper thyroidism is diagnosed by estimating:

(a) T_3 (b) T_4
(c) TSH in plasma (d) All of them

71. Hypothyroidism is characterized by:

(a) Reduced BMR (b) Slow heart rate
(c) Weight gain (d) All of them

72. Hypothyroidism in children is associated with:

(a) Physical retardation (b) Mental retardation
(c) Both (a) and (b) (d) None of them

73. The hydroxylation of dopamine forms nor-epinephrine in presence of:

(a) Ascrobic acid (b) Oxygen
(c) Both (a) and (b) (d) None of them

74. Methylation of noradrenaline leads to the formation of:

(a) Adrenaline (b) Epinephrine
(c) Nor-epinephrine (d) None of them

75. An important derivative of histidine is the local hormone named:

(a) Adrenaline (b) Nor-adrenaline

(c) Histamine (d) Epinephrine

76. Serotonin is converted to 5-hydroxyindol acetic acid by the enzyme:

(a) Phosphofructokinase (b) Monoamine oxidase

(c) Pepsin (d) None of them

77. The end product of serotonin catabolism is:

(a) Tyrosine (b) 5-hydroxyindoleacetic acid

(c) Dopamine (d) None of them

78. Serotonin, which is derived from tryptophan, functions in the central pathways of the brain as a:

(a) Neurotransmitter (b) Inhibitor of gluconeogenesis

(c) Inhibitor of TCA cycle (d) Accelerator of glycolysis

79. In addition to its localization in the brain, serotonin also exists in high concentration in:

(a) Liver (b) Kidney

(c) Pancreas (d) Gastrointestinal tract

80. Another name of serotonin is:

(a) 5-hydroxytryptamine (b) 5-hydroxy tryptophan

(c) Morphine (d) Indoleacetic acid

81. Insulin secretion is reduced by:

(a) Vasectomy (b) Cholecystectomy

(c) Vagatomy (d) Nephrectomy

82. Normal pancreas can store insulin nearly:

(a) 150 units (b) 200 units

(c) 250 units (d) 300 units

83. Insulin can be inactivated by all except:

(a) Lipolytic enzymes (b) EDTA

(c) Folic acid (d) All of them

84. Insulin hormone has a molecular weight of:

(a) 5,000 (b) 5,700

(c) 5,734 (d) 5,834

85. Normal requirement of insulin per day by a normal man is about:

(a) 100 units (b) 150 units

(c) 50 units (d) 250 units

86. An intra sulphide bridge between two amino acids also occurs in the A polypeptide chain of insulin hormone:

(a) Between 6th and 10th (b) Between 6th and 11th

(c) Between 6th and 12th (d) Between 6th and 13th

87. The two polypeptide chains (A and B) of insulin hormone remain linked to each other with the help of disulphide bridges at positions:

(a) 7 (A Chain)–5 (B Chain) and 20 (A Chain)–7 (B Chain)

(b) 7 (A Chain)–3 (B Chain) and 20 (A Chain)–8 (B Chain)

(c) 7 (A Chain)–7 (B Chain) and 20 (A Chain)–9 (B Chain)

(d) 7 (A Chain)–8 (B Chain) and 20 (A Chain)–20 (B Chain)

88. Crystalline insulin was isolated from pancreas in 1926 by:

(a) Abel (b) Fischer

(c) Benedict (d) Henry

89. Level of insulin in the serum in fasting state of a normal person:

(a) 20-50 p mol/Litre (b) 43-98 p mol/Litre

(c) 43-186 p mol/Litre (d) 75-150 p mol/Litre

90. Amino acid sequence of insulin was established in 1953 by:

(a) Smith (b) Sanger

(c) Mitchell (d) Jacob

91. Traces of which metal are required for the crystallization of insulin:

(a) Cobalt (b) Aluminium

(c) Zinc (d) Iron

92. Insulin hormone consists of how many amino acids in its structure:

(a) 49 (b) 50

(c) 51 (d) 52

93. Insulin hormone consists of how many polypeptide chains in its structure:

(a) 2 (b) 3

(c) 4 (d) 5

94. A and B polypeptide chains of insulin hormone consists of how many amino acids in them:

(a) 20 and 31
(b) 21 and 30
(c) 22 and 29
(d) 23 and 28

95. Neurotransmitters are similar to hormones in:

(a) Synthesis
(b) Transport
(c) Mechanism of action
(d) All of them

96. From anterior pituitary, the following hormones are originated:

(a) Lutenizing hormone
(b) Chorionic gonadotropin
(c) Prolactin
(d) All of them

97. The hormones that inhibit adenylate cyclase activity are:

(a) Angiotensin II
(b) α_2- adrenergics
(c) Somatostatin
(d) All of them

98. Atriopeptins – small group of peptides, synthesized by cardiac atrial tissue cause:

(a) Vasodilation
(b) Diuresis
(c) Inhibit aldosterone secretion
(d) All of them

99. Thyrotropin-releasing hormone (TRH) is a tripeptide consists of:

(a) Glutamate derivative
(b) Histidine
(c) Proline
(d) All of them

100. Increased protein bound iodine (PBI) is associated with:

(a) Hyperthyroidism
(b) Hypothyroidism
(c) Both (a) and (b)
(d) None of them

101. Important neurotransmitters in the brain and autonomic nervous system are:

(a) Dopamine
(b) Nor-epinephrine
(c) Both (a) and (b)
(d) None of them

102. Catecholamines increase:

(a) Cardiac output
(b) Blood pressure
(c) Oxygen consumption
(d) All of them

103. The study of receptors is based on the response to:

(a) Agonists
(b) Antagonists
(c) Both (a) and (b)
(d) None of them

104. The steroid sex hormones are responsible for:

(a) Growth

(b) Development

(c) Maintenance and regulation of reproductive system

(d) All of them

105. Primary hypogonadism occurs due to deficiency in ovarian function causing:

(a) Decreased ovulation

(b) Insufficient hormone production

(c) Either (a) or (b)

(d) Neither (a) or (b)

106. The diagnosis of pheochromocytomas is possible only when there is excessive production of:

(a) Epinephrine (b) Nor-epinephrine

(c) Both (a) and (b) (d) None of them

107. Glucocorticoids promote:

(a) Transcription (b) Protein biosynthesis

(c) Both (a) and (b) (d) None of them

108 For the synthesis of steroid hormones, the enzymes responsible are:

(a) Hydroxylases (b) Dehydrogenases

(c) Isomerases (d) All of them

109. In hypothyroidism, serum cholesterol level is:

(a) Increased (b) Decreased

(c) Remains stable (d) None of them

110. Cretinism in children is associated with:

(a) Physical retardation (b) Mental retardation

(c) Both (a) and (b) (d) None of them

111. Endorphins and enkephalins are the natural analgesics that control:

(a) Pain (b) Emotions

(c) Both (a) and (b) (d) None of them

112. Prolactin is concerned with:

(a) Initiation (b) Maintenance of lactation

(c) Both (a) and (b) (d) None of them

113. Prolactin is also known as:

(a) Lactogenic hormone
(b) Luteotropic hormone
(c) Mammotropin hormone
(d) All of them

114. Somatostation is the first polypeptide which was expressed in *E.coli* as a part of the fusion peptide which inhibited the secretion of:

(a) Growth hormone
(b) Glucagon
(c) Insulin
(d) All of them

115. β- endorphin growth hormone, a long neuropeptide having amino acid in number:

(a) 10
(b) 20
(c) 30
(d) 40

Answer Key

1	(d)	26	(b)	51	(d)	76	(b)
2	(b)	27	(c)	52	(d)	77	(b)
3	(c)	28	(a)	53	(c)	78	(a)
4	(a)	29	(a)	54	(d)	79	(d)
5	(a)	30	(c)	55	(c)	80	(a)
6	(b)	31	(a)	56	(c)	81	(c)
7	(a)	32	(c)	57	(d)	82	(c)
8	(a)	33	(c)	58	(c)	83	(d)
9	(b)	34	(c)	59	(a)	84	(c)
10	(a)	35	(c)	60	(d)	85	(c)
11	(a)	36	(d)	61	(c)	86	(b)
12	(b)	37	(a)	62	(d)	87	(c)
13	(b)	38	(b)	63	(c)	88	(a)
14	(b)	39	(a)	64	(a)	89	(c)
15	(d)	40	(d)	65	(d)	90	(b)
16	(b)	41	(c)	66	(c)	91	(c)
17	(c)	42	(d)	67	(c)	92	(c)
18	(a)	43	(d)	68	(d)	93	(a)
19	(b)	44	(a)	69	(d)	94	(b)
20	(a)	45	(a)	70	(d)	95	(d)
21	(b)	46	(a)	71	(d)	96	(d)
22	(a)	47	(c)	72	(c)	97	(d)
23	(a)	48	(c)	73	(c)	98	(d)
24	(a)	49	(d)	74	(a)	99	(d)
25	(d)	50	(c)	75	(c)	100	(a)

101	**(c)**	**105**	**(c)**	**109**	**(a)**	**113**	**(d)**
102	**(d)**	**106**	**(c)**	**110**	**(c)**	**114**	**(d)**
103	**(c)**	**107**	**(c)**	**111**	**(c)**	**115**	**(c)**
104	**(d)**	**108**	**(d)**	**112**	**(c)**		

Chapter 10

Biological Oxidation

1. **Enzymes involving transfer of electron of the hydrogen atoms of the substrate to oxygen are known as:**

   (a) Oxygenases (b) Oxidases

   (c) Dehydrogenases (d) Hydroperoxidases

2. **Enzymes which remove hydrogen from the substrate and pass it directly to oxygen are known as:**

   (a) Oxygenases (b) Oxidases

   (c) Aerobic dehydrogenases (d) Anaerobic dehydrogenases

3. **Oxidases are conjugated proteins having the prosthetic group:**

   (a) Magnesium (b) Manganese

   (c) Copper (d) Iron

4. **Aerobic dehydrogenases having the prosthetic group:**

   (a) ATP (b) NAD^+

   (c) FAD^+ (d) $NADP^+$

5. **NADP linked dehydrogenases in the extramitochondria are found to synthesize:**

   (a) Carbohydrates (b) Fatty acids

   (c) Vitamins (d) Urea

6. **When substrates are oxidized through NAD-linked dehydrogenase, P:O ratio is:**
   (a) 1 (b) 2
   (c) 3 (d) 4

7. **The uncoupling agent of oxidative phosphorylation is:**
   (a) Barbiturates (b) Penicillin
   (c) Antimycin A (d) Dicoumarol

8. **The common currency of energy in biological reaction is:**
   (a) AMP (b) ADP
   (c) ATP (d) UDPG

9. **The number of high energy bonds in adenosine triphosphate is:**
   (a) 1 (b) 2
   (c) 3 (d) 0

10. **The structure of co-enzyme Q is very similar to:**
    (a) Vitamin K (b) Vitamin E
    (c) Both (a) and (b) (d) None of them

11. **Site III of respiratory chain is inhibited by:**
    (a) Dimercaprol (b) Antimycin A
    (c) Both (a) and (b) (d) None of them

12. **Name the compound with greatest standard free energy:**
    (a) ATP (b) Phosphocreatine
    (c) Cyclic AMP (d) Phosphoenol pyruvate

13. **One of the following components of ETC possess isoprenoid units:**
    (a) Co-enzyme Q (b) Cytochrome C
    (c) Cytochrome B (d) Non-heme iron

14. **The P:O ratio for the oxidation of $FADH_2$ is:**
    (a) 1 (b) 2
    (c) 3 (d) 4

15. **Inner mitochondrial membrane is impermeable to:**
    (a) H^+ (b) K^+
    (c) OH- (d) All of them

16. ATP synthetase activity is associated with the mitochondrial enzyme complex:

(a) V
(b) III
(c) IV
(d) I

17. The electron transport chain is located in:

(a) Inner mitochondrial membrane
(b) Outer mitochondrial membrane
(c) Both (a) and (b)
(d) None of them

18. Cytochrome oxidase is:

(a) aa_3
(b) a_3
(c) a
(d) None of them

19. Cytochrome oxidase is poisoned by:

(a) Cyanide
(b) Sulphide
(c) Sulphite
(d) Sulphate

20. Phenolase is an enzyme containing:

(a) Cobalt
(b) Iron
(c) Zinc
(d) Copper

21. Monoamine oxidase oxidizes:

(a) Epinephrine
(b) Nor-epinephrine
(c) Glucagon
(d) Glutathione

22. Uricase catalyzes the oxidation of uric acid to:

(a) Carbon dioxide
(b) Ammonia
(c) Glyoxal
(d) Allantoin

23. Xanthine dehydrogenase converts purine bases to:

(a) Uric acid
(b) Hypoxanthine
(c) Xanthine
(d) Urea

24. The endoplasmic reticulum cytochrome:

(a) b
(b) C
(c) a_1
(d) P-450

25. Mono-oxygenases are found in the:

(a) Mitochondria
(b) Microsomes
(c) Nuclei
(d) Cytosol

26. The mitochondrial superoxide dismutase contains:

(a) Mg^{++} (b) Zn^{++}

(c) Mn^{++} (d) Co^{++}

27. The uncoupling agent of oxidative phosphorylation:

(a) Antimycin A (b) Dicoumarol

(c) Barbiturates (d) Penicillin

28. The oxidation and phosphorylation in intact mitochondria is completely blocked by:

(a) Streptomycin (b) Gentamycin

(c) Puromycin (d) Oligomycin

29. The antibiotic piericidin A inhibits the site of respiratory chain:

(a) I (b) II

(c) III (d) All of them

30. When substrates are oxidized through NAD-linked dehydrogenase, the P:O ratio is:

(a) 1 (b) 2

(c) 3 (d) 4

31. The respiratory chain is folded into how many loops (oxidation/ reduction) in the membrane:

(a) 1 (b) 2

(c) 3 (d) 4

32. Actively respiring mitochondria accumulates:

(a) Cations (b) Anions

(c) None of them (d) All of them

33. Cytochrome P450 acts on various:

(a) Carcinogens (b) Pollutants

(c) Both (a) and (b) (d) None of them

34. The various hydroxylases present in adrenal play an important role in the biosynthesis of:

(a) Cholesterol (b) Steroid

(c) Both (a) and (b) (d) None of them

35. Cytochrome C is quite stable to:

(a) Heat (b) Acids

(c) Both (a) and (b) (d) None of them

36. Respiration is totally blocked by:

(a) H_2S (b) CO

(c) Cyanide (d) All of them

37. Site I of respiratory chain is inhibited by:

(a) Amobarbital (b) Piericidin

(c) Fish poison rotenone (d) All of them

38. The reduced form of cytochrome C is:

(a) Autooxidizable (b) Non-autooxidizable

(c) Both (a) and (b) (d) None of them

39. Cytochrome C has a molecular weight of:

(a) 10,000 (b) 12,000

(c) 13,000 (d) 15,000

40. Two cysteine residues of cytochrome C are located at position:

(a) 14 (b) 17

(c) Both (a) and (b) (d) None of them

41. In the adrenal, cytochrome P-450 are found in:

(a) Mitochondria (b) Endoplasmic reticulum

(c) Both (a) and (b) (d) None of them

42. Hydroxylation reactions take place by the enzyme:

(a) Monooxygenases (b) Cytochrome P-450

(c) Both (a) and (b) (d) None of them

43. Many drugs are metabolized in the liver by a system that utilizes:

(a) Hemoprotein (b) Cytochrome P-450

(c) Heme (d) All of them

44. Mitochondria are generally impermeable to:

(a) Protein (b) Other ions

(c) Both (a) and (b) (d) None of them

45. A single loop of respiratory chain consists of:

(a) Hydrogen carrier (b) Electron carrier

(c) Both (a) and (b) (d) None of them

46. Redox potential is a quantitative measure of the tendency of redox pair to:

(a) Loose electrons
(b) Gain electrons
(c) Either (a) or (b)
(d) Neither (a) or (b)

47. The high energy compound is:

(a) UDPG
(b) ATP
(c) ADP
(d) Arginine phosphate

48. Oligomycin prevents:

(a) Mitochondrial oxidation
(b) Phosphorylation
(c) Both (a) and (b)
(d) None of them

49. Various oxidations occur in other part of cell except mitochondria and liberate:

(a) Heat
(b) Energy
(c) Both (a) and (b)
(d) None of them

50. In the endoplasmic reticulum of human liver isoforms of cytochrome P-450 present are:

(a) Six
(b) Five
(c) Four
(d) Two

Answer Key

1	(b)	14	(b)	27	(b)	40	(c)
2	(c)	15	(d)	28	(d)	41	(c)
3	(c)	16	(a)	29	(a)	42	(c)
4	(c)	17	(a)	30	(c)	43	(d)
5	(b)	18	(a)	31	(c)	44	(c)
6	(c)	19	(a)	32	(a)	45	(c)
7	(d)	20	(d)	33	(c)	46	(c)
8	(c)	21	(a)	34	(c)	47	(a)
9	(b)	22	(d)	35	(c)	48	(c)
10	(c)	23	(a)	36	(d)	49	(a)
11	(c)	24	(d)	37	(d)	50	(a)
12	(d)	25	(b)	38	(b)		
13	(a)	26	(c)	39	(c)		

Chapter 11

Digestion and Absorption

1. **The dietary food which is not in the proper form for absorption into the blood is:**
   (a) Monosaccharides
   (b) Polysaccharides
   (c) Minerals
   (d) Vitamins in free state

2. **Mastication of food performs following functions:**
   (a) Breaks down food into small pieces
   (b) Helps in swallowing solid food
   (c) Increases surface area of food for better contact with digestive enzymes
   (d) All of them

3. **Digestion of food starts in:**
   (a) Mouth
   (b) Stomach
   (c) Small intestine
   (d) Large intestine

4. **The pH of the freshly secreted saliva is about:**
   (a) 4.3-5.8
   (b) 6.3-6.8
   (c) 7.0
   (d) 7.3-8.8

5. **Salivary amylase is mainly secreted by:**
   (a) Parotid glands
   (b) Sub-lingual glands
   (c) Sub maxillary glands
   (d) None of them

6. **Salivary amylase becomes inactive at pH:**
   (a) 6.0
   (b) 5.0
   (c) 4.0
   (d) None of them

7. **Hydrochloric acid of the gastric juice is secreted mainly by the:**
   (a) Cheif of cells of gastric glands
   (b) Parietal cells of gastric tubules
   (c) Columnar cells of the neck of gastric gland
   (d) None of them

8. **Ordinarily, the amount of secretion of gastric juice by an adult per 24 hours is:**
   (a) 1-2 L
   (b) 2-3 L
   (c) 3-4 L
   (d) 4-5L

9. **Gastric juice of newly born infants contains:**
   (a) Only pepsin
   (b) Only rennin
   (c) More amount of rennin
   (d) Equal amounts of pepsin and rennin

10. **The percentage of organic materials in gastric juice is about:**
    (a) 0.1
    (b) 0.2
    (c) 0.4
    (d) 0.8

11. **The amount of HCl in gastric secretion is increased under the stimulation of:**
    (a) Protamine
    (b) Prolamine
    (c) Histamine
    (d) Albumin

12. **The free HCl acidity and the total acidity of the normal gastric juice, respectively is:**
    (a) 50 and 60
    (b) 60 and 50
    (c) 40 and 50
    (d) 40 and 60

13. **When HCl level in gastric juice is nearly zero, condition is known as:**
    (a) Hyperacidity
    (b) Hypoacidity
    (c) Achlorhydria
    (d) None of them

14. **Pepsin is active in:**
    (a) Acidic medium
    (b) Neutral medium
    (c) Alkaline medium
    (d) None of them

15. Pepsin has a molecular weight of:
(a) 31600 (b) 32700
(c) 33300 (d) 34400

16. Rennin changes the casein of milk to paracasein in presence of:
(a) Na^+ (b) K^+
(c) Ca^{2+} (d) Mn^{2+}

17. Topfer' indicator is used for determining:
(a) Free HCl (b) Free and combined HCl
(c) Combined HCl (d) Organic acids

18. The pH value of pancreatic juice lies in the range of:
(a) 1.5-2.5 (b) 4.5-5.5
(c) 7.5-8.2 (d) 8.5-9.5

19. The number of amino acid molecules in a trypsin molecule is:
(a) 123 (b) 223
(c) 232 (d) 322

20. Trypsin attacks peptide linkages containing the amino acid residue:
(a) Glycine (b) Phenylalanine
(c) Tyrosine (d) Arginine

21. Chymotyrpsin attacks peptide linkages containing the amino acid residue:
(a) Glycine (b) Phenylalanine
(c) Leucine (d) Arginine

22. Carboxypeptidase B hydrolyses terminal peptide linkages containing:
(a) Glycine and valine (b) Leucine and isoleucine
(c) Lysine and arginine (d) Serine and tryptophan

23. Collagenase hydrolyses collagen present in:
(a) Milk (b) Soybean
(c) Egg (d) Meat

24. The activity of steapsin is increased by:
(a) Ca^{2+} (b) Soaps
(c) Bile salts (d) All of them

25. Pancreatic juice contains:

(a) Proteolytic enzymes (b) Lipolytic enzymes
(c) Amylolytic enzymes (d) All of them

26. Steapsin is a digestive enzyme concerning the digestion of:

(a) Carbohydrates (b) Lipids
(c) Proteins (d) Nucleic acids

27. The percentage of water in intestinal juice is about:

(a) 95.5 (b) 96.5
(c) 97.5 (d) 98.5

28. The function of enteropeptidase found in intestinal juice is:

(a) To digest proteins (b) To activate trypsinogen
(c) Both (a) and (b) (d) None of them

29. The inorganic substances present in the solids of intestinal juice are nearly:

(a) $1/4^{th}$ (b) 1/2
(c) $1/3^{rd}$ (d) $2/3^{rd}$

30. The pH value of bile lies in the range of:

(a) 5-6.5 (b) 7.0-7.5
(c) 7-8.5 (d) 8.6-9.6

31. The amount of bile secreted by liver daily is:

(a) 200-600ml (b) 500-1000ml
(c) 700-1500ml (d) 800-1800ml

32. The hormone that stimulates the release of bile from gall bladder is:

(a) Insulin (b) Secretin
(c) Hepatocrinin (d) Cholecystokinin

33. Bile acids are derived from the parent acid called:

(a) Cholic acid (b) Cholanic acid
(c) Taurocholic acid (d) Prostanoic acid

34. In bile, bile acids are present as:

(a) Free (b) Conjugates with glycine
(c) Conjugates with taurine (d) Both (a) and (b)

35. Bile acids are produced from cholesterol in:

(a) Intestine (b) Liver

(c) Gall bladder (d) Stomach

36. The percentage of bile salts reabsorbed in the intestine and returned to the liver is:

(a) 70-75 (b) 80-85

(c) 90-95 (d) 100

37. The amount of bile salts that escapes reabsorption in the intestine and thus eliminated in the feces is:

(a) 300mg (b) 500mg

(c) 700mg (d) 1000mg

38. In liver and gall bladder, gallstones are formed when:

(a) The bile acid: cholesterol ratio falls below a critical value

(b) The bile acid: cholesterol ratio increases above a critical level

(c) Both (a) and (b)

(d) None of them

39. Yellow colour of bile is due to:

(a) Biliverdin (b) Bilirubin

(c) Either (a) or (b) (d) Neither (a) or (b)

40. In jaundice excess of bile pigments are accumulated in:

(a) Liver (b) Intestine

(c) Blood (d) Gall bladder

41. The most important organ concerning absorption is:

(a) Stomach (b) Small intestine

(c) Large intestine (d) All the three

42. The carbohydrate that is most easily absorbed is:

(a) Glucose (b) Fructose

(c) Sucrose (d) Galactose

43. Steatorrhoea is a condition in which feces contain large amounts of unabsorbed:

(a) Carbohydrates (b) Fats

(c) Proteins (d) Water

44. Which of the following is a correct statement:

(a) D-and L-isomers of an amino acid are absorbed at the same rate

(b) L-isomer of an amino acid is absorbed more quickly, than the corresponding D-isomer

(c) The D-isomer of an amino acid is absorbed more quickly than the corresponding L-isomer

(d) None of them

45. The important reaction taking place in putrefaction is the:

(a) Decarboxylation of amino acids

(b) Deamination of amino acids

(c) Both (a) and (b)

(d) None of them

46. Indole and skatole, the main fowl smelling compounds of the feces are the degradation products of:

(a) Tyrosine
(b) Tryptophan
(c) Phenylalanine
(d) Cystine

47. The change in colour of adult feces on exposure to air is due to the:

(a) Presence of H_2S in feces

(b) Presence of bilinogens

(c) Presence of bilins

(d) Coversion of bilinogen to bilins

48. Intestinal fermentation is concerned with:

(a) The decomposition of any compound in intestine by bacteria

(b) The decomposition of carbohydrates to organic acids by bacteria

(c) Decomposition of proteins

(d) Decomposition of fats

49. Transport of glucose from lumen to the intestinal mucosal cells is coupled with diffusion of:

(a) Na^+
(b) K^+
(c) Cl^-
(d) HCO_3^-

50. The key enzyme that converts trypsinogen to trypsin is:

(a) Secretin
(b) Chymotrypsin
(c) Elastase
(d) Enteropeptidase

51. The products obtained by the action of pancreatic lipase on triacylglycerols are:

(a) Glycerol and free fatty acids

(b) 1-Acylglycerol and free fatty acids

(c) 2-Acylglycerol and free fatty acids

(d) 3-Acylglycerol and free fatty acids

52. The lipoproteins synthesized in the intestinal mucosal cells from the absorbed lipids are:

(a) High density lipoproteins

(b) Chylomicrons

(c) Low density lipoproteins

(d) Very low density lipoproteins

53. Salivary α-amylase becomes inactive in the stomach due to:

(a) Inactivation by low pH

(b) Degradation by gastric pepsin

(c) Inhibition by Cl^-

(d) Inhibition by peptides

54. Cellulose is not digested in human due to lack of enzyme that hydrolyses:

(a) α-Glycosidic bond (b) β-Glycosidic bond

(c) Both (a) and (b) (d) None of them

55. Trypsin hydrolyses peptide bonds, the carbonyl group of which is contributed by:

(a) Arginine (b) Lysine

(c) Either (a) or (b) (d) None of them

56. The amount of saliva secreted each day in ml:

(a) 600-800 (b) 700-900

(c) 800-1000 (d) 1000-1500

57. The sub-maxillary secretion contains most of the:

(a) Glycoproteins (b) Glycolipids

(c) Both (a) and (b) (d) None of them

58. Saliva contains inorganic materials in per cent:

(a) 0.1 (b) 0.2

(c) 0.3 (d) 0.4

59. The amylase is helped to be stabilized by:

(a) Ca^{++} (b) Mg^{++}

(c) Na^{+} (d) K^{+}

60. The continued gastric secretions regulated by the hormone:

(a) Glucagon (b) Gastrin

(c) Epinephrine (d) ACTH

61. Pepsin converts native protein into:

(a) Proteoses (b) Peptones

(c) Both (a) and (b) (d) None of them

62. Hydrochloric acid secreted by oxyntic cells contain the pH:

(a) 0.5 (b) 0.6

(c) 0.8 (d) 0.9

63. Bile salts help in the absorption of:

(a) Cholesterol (b) Fatty acids

(c) Vitamin D (d) All of them

64. On ordinary diet, the daily amount of secretion of gastric juice by an adult in litres is:

(a) 1-2 (b) 2-3

(c) 3-4 (d) 4-5

65. The intrinsic factor (HCl and mucoproteins) present in the gastric juice helps in the absorption of:

(a) Vitamin B_2 (b) Biotin

(c) Folic acid (d) Vitamin B_{12}

66. Hydrochloric acid stimulates duodenum to liberate:

(a) Secretin (b) Pepsin

(c) Trypsin (d) Enterocrinin

67. Pepsin contains large amount of amino acids:

(a) Neutral (b) Basic

(c) Acidic (d) Sulphur containing

68. Pepsin has a molecular weight of:

(a) 31,600 (b) 32,700

(c) 33,300 (d) 34,400

69. Salivary amylase is acted by:

(a) Na^+ (b) K^+

(c) Cl^- (d) None of them

70. Lipase can act only at the pH:

(a) 3.0 to 4.5 (b) 3.5 to 5.0

(c) 4.0 to 6.0 (d) 5.0 to 7.0

71. Pancreatic juice contains percentage of solids:

(a) 1.6 (b) 1.8

(c) 2.0 (d) 2.2

72. The amount of pancreatic juice secreted each day in ml:

(a) 300-500 (b) 400-600

(c) 500-700 (d) 600-800

73. Carboxypeptidase contains:

(a) Zinc (b) Copper

(c) Manganese (d) Magnesium

74. The mucopolysaccharide present in intrinsic factor contains:

(a) Fucose (b) Hexosamine

(c) Neuraminic acid (d) All of them

75. RNAse and DNAse are capable of cleaving internal:

(a) Phosphodiester bonds (b) Diester bonds

(c) Ester bonds (d) None of them

76. The percentage of solids in intestinal juice is about:

(a) 0.5 (b) 0.1

(c) 1.5 (d) 2.0

77. Bile is produced by:

(a) Liver (b) Gall bladder

(c) Pancreas (d) Intestine

78. Bile formed daily in adult human beings in molecules of about:

(a) 200 to 800 (b) 300 to 1200

(c) 700 to 1500 (d) 800 to 1800

79. Bile acids are synthesized from cholesterol in:

(a) Duodenum (b) Intestine

(c) Gall bladder (d) Liver

80. In human bile, sodium glycocholate is greater than sodium taurocholate by:

(a) Two times (b) Three times

(c) Four times (d) Five times

81. Bile salts activate:

(a) Pancreatic lipase (b) Cholesterol esterase

(c) Both (a) and (b) (d) None of them

82. In obstructive jaundice, bile salts in blood are:

(a) Decreased (b) Highly decreased

(c) Increased (d) Greatly increased

83. The amount of bile salts in mg per day are not absorbed and is eliminated in the feces:

(a) 500 (b) 700

(c) 900 (d) 1200

84. Bile is an important source of:

(a) Acid (b) Alkali

(c) Salt (d) None of them

85. Arginine is decarboxylated by the intestinal bacteria into:

(a) Agmatine (b) Arginamine

(c) Arginatine (d) Argininemine

86. By a series of reactions in the large intestine tryptophan forms:

(a) Indole (b) Methyl indole

(c) Both (a) and (b) (d) None of them

87. In the large intestine, cysteine by a series of transformation forms:

(a) Ethyl mercaptan (b) Methyl mercaptan

(c) H_2S (d) All of them

88. The quantity of ammonia transported from large intestine to the blood is reduced by the antibacterial action of:

(a) Streptomycin (b) Neomycin

(c) Penicillin (d) Chloramphenicol

89. The reduction of biliverdin to urobilinogen takes place in the:

(a) Duodenum (b) Small intestine

(c) Large intestine (d) All of them

90. Cathepsins occur in the:

(a) Mitochondria (b) Cytosol

(c) Nuclei (d) Lysosomes

91. Enterocrinin is released from the:

(a) Duodenal mucosa (b) Pancreas

(c) Large intestine (d) Small intestine

92. The secretion of enterogastrone by the duodenal mucosa is influenced by the dietary:

(a) Carbohydrates (b) Fats

(c) Proteins (d) Minerals

93. Enterogastrin inhibits the secretion of:

(a) HCl (b) Pepsin

(c) Both (a) and (b) (d) None of them

94. Gastrin stimulates the secretion of:

(a) HCl (b) Pepsin

(c) Intrinsic factor (d) All of them

95. In herbivora, the intestinal bacteria also synthesize:

(a) Essential amino acids (b) Vitamins

(c) Both (a) and (b) (d) None of them

96. Initiation of gastric secretion is caused by the mechanism:

(a) Nervous (b) Reflex

(c) Either (a) or (b) (d) Neither (a) or (b)

97. Carbonic anhydrase catalyzes the formation of H_2CO_3 from:

(a) H_2O (b) CO_2

(c) Both (a) and (b) (d) None of them

98. Pepsin converts native proteins into:

(a) Proteoses (b) Peptones

(c) Both (a) and (b) (d) None of them

99. The secretion of pancreatic juice is controlled by the means:

(a) Hormonal (b) Nervous

(c) Both (a) and (b) (d) None of them

100. Pancreatic amylase is an:

(a) α-amylase
(b) Endoamylase
(c) Both (a) and (b)
(d) None of them

101. Mixed gall stones are composed of:

(a) Cholesterol
(b) Bile pigments
(c) Both (a) and (b)
(d) None of them

102. Renal calculi is due to the urine:

(a) Infection
(b) Stagnation
(c) Both (a) and (b)
(d) None of them

103. Lecithin is decomposed to:

(a) Choline
(b) Neurine
(c) Both (a) and (b)
(d) None of them

104. Urate stones are formed due to:

(a) Hyperuricemia
(b) Gout
(c) Both (a) and (b)
(d) None of them

Answer Key

1	(b)	27	(d)	53	(c)	79	(d)
2	(d)	28	(b)	54	(b)	80	(b)
3	(a)	29	(d)	55	(c)	81	(c)
4	(b)	30	(c)	56	(d)	82	(d)
5	(a)	31	(b)	57	(a)	83	(a)
6	(c)	32	(d)	58	(b)	84	(b)
7	(b)	33	(b)	59	(a)	85	(a)
8	(b)	34	(d)	60	(b)	86	(c)
9	(c)	35	(b)	61	(c)	87	(d)
10	(c)	36	(c)	62	(d)	88	(b)
11	(c)	37	(b)	63	(d)	89	(c)
12	(a)	38	(a)	64	(b)	90	(d)
13	(c)	39	(b)	65	(d)	91	(a)
14	(a)	40	(c)	66	(a)	92	(b)
15	(b)	41	(b)	67	(c)	93	(c)
16	(c)	42	(d)	68	(b)	94	(d)
17	(a)	43	(b)	69	(c)	95	(c)
18	(c)	44	(b)	70	(d)	96	(c)
19	(b)	45	(c)	71	(b)	97	(c)
20	(d)	46	(b)	72	(d)	98	(c)
21	(b)	47	(d)	73	(a)	99	(c)
22	(c)	48	(b)	74	(d)	100	(c)
23	(d)	49	(a)	75	(a)	101	(c)
24	(d)	50	(a)	76	(c)	102	(c)
25	(d)	51	(b)	77	(a)	103	(c)
26	(b)	52	(d)	78	(b)	104	(c)

Chapter 12

Hemoglobin, Porphyrin and Bile Pigments

1. **Hemoglobin contains the number of g atoms of iron in ferrous state:**
   (a) 1 (b) 2
   (c) 3 (d) 4

2. **The molecular weight of hemoglobin is:**
   (a) 44450 (b) 54450
   (c) 64450 (d) 84450

3. **The total number of amino acids in globin is:**
   (a) 544 (b) 554
   (c) 564 (d) 574

4. **The iron of heme is co-ordinated in β-chains at positions:**
   (a) 43 and 72 (b) 53 and 82
   (c) 63 and 92 (d) 73 and 102

5. **Porphyrin rings are cyclic compounds composed of pyrrole rings:**
   (a) 4 (b) 3
   (c) 2 (d) 5

6. **The characteristic red colour of hemoglobin is due to:**
   (a) Heme (b) α-globin
   (c) β-globin (d) All of them

7. **The number of heme groups present in myoglobin:**
   (a) 1 (b) 2
   (c) 3 (d) 4

8. **The compound that facilitates the release of O_2 from oxyhemoglobin:**
   (a) 2,3-Biphosphoglycerate (b) H^+
   (c) Cl^- (d) All of them

9. **Name the amino acid that directly participates in the synthesis of heme:**
   (a) Methionine (b) Aspartate
   (c) Glycine (d) Tryptophan

10. **The product formed when heme oxygenase cleaves heme:**
    (a) Biliverdin (b) Bilirubin
    (c) Both (a) and (b) (d) None of them

11. **The porphyrins are found in nature in which various chains are substituted for the hydrogenation no:**
    (a) 2 (b) 4
    (c) 6 (d) 8

12. **A porphyrin with a completely symmetrical arrangement of the substituent's is classified as porphyrin of:**
    (a) Type I (b) Type II
    (c) Type III (d) All of them

13. **In the biosynthesis of porphyrins the activation of glycine needs the coenzyme:**
    (a) NAD^+ (b) B_6-PO_4
    (c) FAD^+ (d) ATP

14. **The anemia has been observed in the deficiency of vitamin:**
    (a) Biotin (b) Inositol
    (c) Niacin (d) Pantothenic acid

15. **Catalases contain the number of gram atoms of iron per mole:**
    (a) 1 (b) 2
    (c) 3 (d) 4

16. The colour of cyanomethemoglobin is:

(a) Yellow (b) Pink

(c) Brown (d) Bright red

17. Methemoglobin can be reduced to hemoglobin by:

(a) Removal of hydrogen (b) Vitamin

(c) Glutathione (d) Creatinine

18. Methemoglobin is formed as a result of oxidation of hemoglobin by oxidizing agent:

(a) Oxygen of air (b) Hydrogen peroxide

(c) Potassium ferricyanide (d) Potassium permanganate

19. One molecule of hemoglobin contains histidine residues:

(a) 5 (b) 15

(c) 25 (d) 35

20. Carboxyhemoglobin is formed by:

(a) CO (b) CO_2

(c) HCO_3 (d) HCN

21. Hemoglobin takes up the number of oxygen molecules:

(a) 1 (b) 2

(c) 4 (d) 6

22. The two α-chains of globin have identical amino acid composition of:

(a) 111 (b) 121

(c) 131 (d) 141

23. The globin of hemoglobin is a protein composed of closely packed polypeptide chains of:

(a) 6 parallel layers (b) 4 parallel layers

(c) 3 parallel layers (d) 2 parallel layers

24. Heme is synthesized by the incorporation of ferrous ion into protoporphyrin III being catalyzed by the enzyme:

(a) Ferro-oxidase (b) Ferro-reductase

(c) Ferro-chelatase (d) None of them

25. Under optimal conditions one gram of hemoglobin can carry oxygen in ml:

(a) 1.0 (b) 1.14

(c) 1.24 (d) 1.34

26. The dipyrrole compounds are of two types:

(a) A and B (b) B and C

(c) A and C (d) B and D

27. A type III porphyrin results with the condensation of the components:

(a) Two of the A (b) One A and one B

(c) Two of the B (d) One A and one C

28. The enzyme coproporphyrinogen oxidase is able to act on copro-porpyrinogen:

(a) Type I (b) Type II

(c) Type III (d) All of them

29. In mammalian liver the reaction of conversion of coproporphyrinogen to protoporphyrin requires:

(a) Molecular oxygen (b) Water

(c) ATP (d) B_6-PO_4

30. Cytochrome oxidases can carry the type of reaction:

(a) Electron transfer (b) Oxygen transfer

(c) Mixed function oxidation (d) All of them

31. For the formation of abnormal hemoglobin from normal hemoglobin, acidic amino acid is replaced by a:

(a) Basic amino acid (b) Neutral amino acid

(c) Either (a) or (b) (d) Neither (a) or (b)

32. In hemoglobin-S sickle cell anemia develops and RBC becomes:

(a) Long (b) Boat shaped

(c) Both (a) and (b) (d) None of them

33. The abnormality of hemoglobin M is found in α-chain, the histidine residues in 58 and 87 position are replaced by:

(a) Tyrosine (b) Tryptophan

(c) Proline (d) None of them

34. Trypsin splits peptides in hemoglobin at the points, where the following occurs:

(a) Lysine (b) Arginine

(c) Both (a) and (b) (d) None of them

35. Methemoglobin is the hemoglobin of type:

(a) Oxidized
(b) Reduced
(c) Both (a) and (b)
(d) None of them

36. Cyanosis develops when the concentration of methemoglobin is:

(a) 3g/100ml blood
(b) 6g/100ml blood
(c) 9g/100ml blood
(d) None of them

37. Erythropoetic porphyria has got tendency to:

(a) Hemolysis
(b) Defective erythropoieis
(c) Both (a) and (b)
(d) None of them

38. In erythropoietic protoporphyria, there is increased:

(a) Protoporphyrin
(b) Uroporphyrin
(c) Both (a) and (b)
(d) None of them

39. Hereditary coproporphyria causes increased urinary output of:

(a) Porphobilinogen
(b) ALA
(c) Both (a) and (b)
(d) None of them

40. Iron is bound to the nitrogen atom of pyrrole ring in:

(a) Ferrous state
(b) Ferric state
(c) Neutral state
(d) None of them

41. The globin of hemoglobin is composed of how many parallel layers of closely packed polypeptide chains?

(a) 4
(b) 3
(c) 2
(d) 5

42. The protoporphyrin yields bilirubin:

(a) 300mg
(b) 400mg
(c) 200mg
(d) 100mg

43. Sickle cells cause:

(a) Hemolytic anemia
(b) Jaundice
(c) Both (a) and (b)
(d) None of them

44. Persons suffering from sickle cell anemia show an increased resistance to:

(a) Malaria
(b) Salmonella
(c) Both (a) and (b)
(d) None of them

45. Bilirubin is formed from biliverdin by bilirubin reductase in presence of:

(a) $NADP^+$
(b) NAD^+
(c) Both (a) and (b)
(d) None of them

46. Acute intermittent porphyria causes periodic attacks of abdominal pain which is associated with:

(a) Fever
(b) Leukocytosis
(c) Both (a) and (b)
(d) None of them

47. Porphyrias are of the types:

(a) Congenital
(b) Acquired
(c) Both (a) and (b)
(d) None of them

48. The oxidation of ferrous ion to ferric iron in hemoglobin results in the formation of:

(a) Oxyhemoglobin
(b) Myoglobin
(c) Methemoglobin
(d) None of them

49. Sickling of RBC in sickle cell anemia is due to the polymerization of:

(a) Oxyhemoglobin
(b) Deoxyhemoglobin
(c) Myoglobin
(d) None of them

50. In obstructive jaundice, the obstruction may be caused by:

(a) Gall stones
(b) Tumors
(c) Both (a) and (b)
(d) None of them

Answer Key

1	(d)	14	(d)	27	(b)	40	(a)
2	(c)	15	(d)	28	(c)	41	(a)
3	(d)	16	(d)	29	(a)	42	(a)
4	(c)	17	(b)	30	(d)	43	(c)
5	(a)	18	(c)	31	(c)	44	(c)
6	(a)	19	(d)	32	(c)	45	(c)
7	(a)	20	(a)	33	(a)	46	(c)
8	(d)	21	(c)	34	(c)	47	(c)
9	(c)	22	(d)	35	(a)	48	(c)
10	(a)	23	(b)	36	(a)	49	(b)
11	(d)	24	(c)	37	(c)	50	(c)
12	(a)	25	(a)	38	(c)		
13	(b)	26	(a)	39	(c)		

Chapter 13

Blood, Lymph and Cerebrospinal Fluid

1. **Blood is classified into four main groups on the basis of the nature of:**
   (a) Erythrocytes (b) Leucocytes
   (c) Thrombocytes (d) All the three
2. **Blood containing no agglutinogen (antigen) in red cells is said to belong to which group?**
   (a) a (b) b
   (c) AB (d) O
3. **Which antibody is found in the blood group O?**
   (a) Anti A (b) Anti b
   (c) Both (a) and (b) (d) None of them
4. **The main amino acid present in blood proteins is:**
   (a) Histidine (b) Lysine
   (c) Threonine (d) All the three
5. **Cellular fraction of blood in volume per cent is:**
   (a) 40 (b) 45
   (c) 55 (d) 60

6. **The non-diffusible substance present in plasma is:**
   (a) Urea (b) Vitamins
   (c) Hormones (d) Proteins

7. **Which constituent is present in the largest amount in blood?**
   (a) Plasma proteins (b) Hemoglobin
   (c) Glucose (d) Urea

8. **Condition in which leukocyte count is below normal is known as:**
   (a) Leucocytosis (b) Leucopemia
   (c) Leucopenia (d) None of them

9. **Purpurea hemorrhagia is characterized by:**
   (a) Bleeding from mucous membrane (b) Appearance of black and blue spots
   (c) Both (a) and (b) (d) None of them

10. **Which one of the following is formed element of blood:**
    (a) Erythrocytes (b) Leucocytes
    (c) Thrombocytes (d) All of three

11. **Hemolysis of blood is caused by:**
    (a) Quinine (b) Ether
    (c) Both (a) and (b) (d) None of them

12. **The commonest Rh antigen is:**
    (a) A (b) B
    (c) D (d) AB

13. **Anemia is characterized by the following points:**
    (a) Decreased number of red cells
    b) Decreased percentage of hemoglobin
    (c) Both (a) and (b)
    (d) None of them

14. **Production of thrombin from prothrombin requires:**
    (a) Thromboplastin (b) Ca^{2+}
    (c) Both (a) and (b) (d) None of them

15. **The normal osmotic pressure of blood is equal to:**
    (a) 0.915% NaCl (b) 0.925% NaCl
    (c) 0.945% NaCl (d) 0.955% NaCl

16. The substance almost entirely confirmed in corpuscles is:

(a) Sodium (b) Calcium

(c) Potassium (d) Magnesium

17. The normal concentration of serum albumin in g per cent by precipitation method is:

(a) 4.5 (b) 5.0

(c) 5.2 (d) 5.4

18. The normal concentration of serum globulin in g per 100ml by precipitation method is:

(a) 2.0 (b) 2.5

(c) 2.9 (d) 3.2

19. Serum β-globulin normal concentration in g per cent is:

(a) 0.82 (b) 0.85

(c) 0.91 (d) 0.95

20. The normal concentration of α_1-globulin in g per cent is:

(a) 0.32 (b) 0.35

(c) 0.38 (d) 0.42

21. Fibrinogen is precipitated by half saturation with:

(a) Ammonium sulphate (b) Barium sulphate

(c) Calcium sulphate (d) Magnesium sulphate

22. Which of the immunoglobulins constitute the largest portion of γ-globulin:

(a) IgA (b) IgG

(c) IgM (d) IgD

23. Foreign bodies entering the body are known as:

(a) Antibodies (b) Antigens

(c) Antibiotics (d) Immunobodies

24. Which one is the natural anticoagulant:

(a) Sodium oxalate (b) Potassium oxalate

(c) Heparin (d) Ammonium oxalate

25. Serum albumin has the molecular weight:

(a) 69000Da (b) 44000Da

(c) 1,50,000Da (d) 6,000Da

26. Immunoglobulin M has molecular weight of:

(a) 900kDa (b) 1000kDa

(c) 1500kDa (d) 600kDa

27. Immunoglobulin M accounts for:

(a) 5-10% (b) 10-20%

(c) 20-40% (d) 0-5%

28. Hemophilia A is due to the deficiency of clotting factor:

(a) X (b) V

(c) VIII (d) II

29. Plasma albumin performs the following functions:

(a) Osmotic (b) Transport

(c) Nutritive (d) All of them

30. The immunoglobulin present in most abundant quantity:

(a) IgG (b) IgA

(c) IgM (d) IgE

31. Name the immunoglobulin involved in body allergic reactions:

(a) IgA (b) IgE

(c) IgD (d) IgM

32. The following anticoagulant binds with Ca^{2+} and prevents blood clotting:

(a) Heparin (b) Oxalate

(c) Protein (d) All of them

33. The immunoglobulin that can cross the placenta and transfer the mother's immunity to the developing fetus:

(a) IgG (b) IgM

(c) IgE (d) None of them

34. The immunoglobulin that can bind with most cells and release histamine:

(a) IgE (b) IgG

(c) Both (a) and (b) (d) None of them

35. The patients of sickle cell anemia are resistant to:

(a) Filaria (b) Malaria

(c) Diabetes (d) Trypanosomiasis

36. Cytochrome oxidases can carry the type of reactions:

(a) Oxygen transfer (b) Mixed function oxidation
(c) Electron transfer (d) All of them

37. Plasma fraction of blood in volume per cent:

(a) 40 (b) 45
(c) 50 (d) All of them

38. The diffusible constituents of plasma:

(a) Uric acid (b) Vitamins
(c) Hormones (d) All of them

39. The catabolic products of diffusible constituents of plasma:

(a) Uric acid (b) Creatinine
(c) Both (a) and (b) (d) None of them

40. The normal concentration of fibrinogen of blood per 100ml:

(a) 0.2-0.6 grams (b) 0.4-0.8 grams
(c) 0.6-1.0 grams (d) 0.8-1.2 grams

41. The normal level of free fatty acids in blood per 100ml:

(a) 110-400mg (b) 120-450mg
(c) 140-480mg (d) 150-500mg

42. The normal blood total lipids concentration in mg/100ml:

(a) 500-750 (b) 550-800
(c) 570-820 (d) 600-850

43. The normal level of bilirubin in serum in mg/100ml:

(a) 0.1-0.4 (b) 0.2-0.9
(c) 0.3-1.2 (d) 0.4-1.5

44. The normal concentration of serum lactate dehydrogenase/L:

(a) 50-100 I.U. (b) 60-120 I.U
(c) 80-150 I.U. (d) 90-200 I.U.

45. The normal level of NPN of blood in mg per cent:

(a) 10-25 (b) 15-35
(c) 20-40 (d) 25-45

46. The ear vein can be used for blood collection in:

(a) Cat (b) Pig
(c) Dog (d) All of them

47. The substances circulating in blood:

(a) Enzymes (b) Vitamins
(c) Hormones (d) All of them

48. Plasma contains the solids in per cent:

(a) 7 to 8 (b) 8 to 9
(c) 9 to 10 (d) 10 to 12

49. The plasma proteins are separated by:

(a) Salt precipitation (b) Electrophoresis
(c) Immuno electrophoresis (d) All of them

50. The number of amino acids arranged in a single peptide chain constituting albumin are:

(a) 580 (b) 600
(c) 610 (d) 620

51. Metalloprotein concentration is reduced in:

(a) Pernicious anemia (b) Chronic infections
(c) Liver diseases (d) All of them

52. Serum albumin concentration decreases in:

(a) Severe protein deficiency (b) Liver diseases
(c) Nephritis (d) All of them

53. Leucocytes contain:

(a) Proteins (b) Nucleoproteins
(c) Fats (d) All of them

54. Blood platelets contain large amount of:

(a) Catecholamines (b) Serotonin
(c) Histamine (d) All of them

55. Thrombin consists of number of polypeptide chains:

(a) 1 (b) 2
(c) 3 (d) 4

56. Some glycoproteins have specific binding function for:

(a) Thyroxine (b) Cortisol

(c) Both (a) and (b) (d) None of them

57. Metalloprotein concentration is increased in:

(a) Iron deficiency (b) Pregnancy

(c) Either (a) or (b) (d) None of them

58. The normal concentration of protein bound iodine of blood per 100ml is:

(a) 2-6μg (b) 4-8μg

(c) 6-10μg (d) 8-12μg

59. The normal concentration of pyruvic acid in blood in mg per cent.:

(a) 0.7-2.0 (b) 0.8-2.2

(c) 1.0-2.5 (d) 1.5-3.0

60. Human blood is thicker than water by the number of times:

(a) 2 (b) 3

(c) 4 (d) 5

61. The human plasma proteins are a mixture of:

(a) Simple proteins (b) Glycoproteins

(c) Lipoproteins (d) All of them

62. β-globulin contains:

(a) Siderophilin (b) Ceruloplasmin

(c) Both (a) and (b) (d) None of them

63. The substance which contains more than 4% hexosamine are designated as:

(a) Glycoproteins (b) Mucoproteins

(c) Both (a) and (b) (d) None of them

64. The minor blood groups are:

(a) M (b) N

(c) Rh (d) All of them

65. Thrombin consists of numbers of polypeptide chains:

(a) 1 (b) 2

(c) 3 (d) 4

66. The total value of C.S.F. in an adult is about:

(a) 130ml (b) 140ml
(c) 150ml (d) 160ml

67. In the fasting adult, sugar in C.S.F. in mg per 100ml is:

(a) 40-60 (b) 50-85
(c) 0-110 (d) 90-130

68. In meningitis, sugar content of C.S.F. is:

(a) Decreased (b) Increased
(c) Remains same (d) None of them

69. In tuberculosis meningitis, the chloride in C.S.F. is:

(a) Reduced (b) Increased
(c) Unchanged (d) None of them

70. Increased level of calcium in C.S.F. is observed in all cases of:

(a) Meningitis (b) Epidemic encephalitis
(c) Both (a) and (b) (d) None of them

71. In malignant brain tumors, isomerase activity of C.S.F. is:

(a) Increased (b) Decreased
(c) Remains unchanged (d) None of them

72. In myxedema, the protein content of C.S.F. is:

(a) Increased (b) Decreased
(c) Unaltered (d) None of them

73. The ratio between albumin and globulin in lymph and plasma is:

(a) Same (b) Different
(c) Both (a) and (b) (d) None of them

74. Antithrombin III has the activity of type:

(a) Exogenous (b) Endogenous
(c) Both (a) and (b) (d) None of them

75. White thrombus is composed of:

(a) Platelets (b) Fibrin
(c) Both (a) and (b) (d) None of them

76. Universal donors are the persons having group:

(a) A (b) B

(c) O (d) None of them

77. Blood platelets are:

(a) Nucleated (b) Unnucleated

(c) Simple (d) None of them

78. Fibrinogen is highly elongated having axial ratio of about:

(a) 20 :1 (b) 10 :1

(c) 30 :1 (d) 40 :1

79. Heparin has got disadvantages:

(a) May cause clumping of WBC (b) Unsuitable for smears

(c) Expensive (d) All of them

80. Defibrinated blood is a mixture of:

(a) Blood cells (b) Serum

(c) Both (a) and (b) (d) None of them

81. α_1-globulins are several complex proteins containing:

(a) Carbohydrates (b) Lipids

(c) Both (a) and (b) (d) None of them

82. Immunoglobulins having antibody activity:

(a) α-globulins (b) β-globulins

(c) γ-globulins (d) None of them

83. The viscosity of blood is affected by the change in number of:

(a) Red cells (b) White cells

(c) Either (a) or (b) (d) Neither (a) or (b)

84. In strenuous exercise osmotic pressure of blood is:

(a) Increased (b) Decreased

(c) Remains same (d) None of them

85. The volume of blood in adult is about:

(a) 3 Litres (b) 5 Litres

(c) 6 Litres (d) 7 Litres

86. Which one of the following is false:

(a) Man has a lower ESR then woman

(b) Newborns have the lowest ESR

(c) The lower the red cell numbers, the greater the ESR

(d) None of them

87. Mainly globulins are responsible for blood viscosity due to:

(a) Large molecular size
(b) Asymmetry in structure
(c) Both (a) and (b)
(d) None of them

88. ESR depends on the relative concentration of:

(a) Fibrinogen
(b) γ_2 globulin
(c) γ globulin
(d) All of them

89. In the process of blood coagulation, following participates:

(a) Prothrombin
(b) Fibrinogen
(c) Enzymes
(d) All of them

90. Clinical symptoms of acute intermittent porphyria are:

(a) Vomiting
(b) Constipation
(c) Neurologic disturbances
(d) All of them

Answer Key

1	(a)	24	(c)	47	(d)	70	(c)
2	(d)	25	(a)	48	(b)	71	(a)
3	(c)	26	(a)	49	(d)	72	(a)
4	(d)	27	(a)	50	(c)	73	(c)
5	(b)	28	(c)	51	(d)	74	(c)
6	(d)	29	(d)	52	(a)	75	(c)
7	(b)	30	(a)	53	(d)	76	(c)
8	(c)	31	(b)	54	(d)	77	(b)
9	(c)	32	(b)	55	(b)	78	(a)
10	(d)	33	(a)	56	(c)	79	(d)
11	(c)	34	(a)	57	(c)	80	(c)
12	(c)	35	(b)	58	(b)	81	(c)
13	(c)	36	(d)	59	(a)	82	(c)
14	(c)	37	(b)	60	(d)	83	(c)
15	(c)	38	(c)	61	(d)	84	(a)
16	(c)	39	(c)	62	(c)	85	(b)
17	(a)	40	(a)	63	(b)	86	(d)
18	(b)	41	(d)	64	(d)	87	(c)
19	(c)	42	(c)	65	(b)	88	(d)
20	(d)	43	(a)	66	(a)	89	(d)
21	(a)	44	(d)	67	(b)	90	(d)
22	(b)	45	(b)	68	(a)		
23	(b)	46	(d)	69	(a)		

Chapter 14

Biological Membrane

1. **Membranes are composed of:**
   (a) Lipids (b) Proteins
   (c) Carbohydrates (d) All of them
2. **Membranes carry out specific functions of:**
   (a) Organelle (b) Cell
   (c) Organism (d) All of them
3. **The selective permeabilities of membrane are regulated by:**
   (a) Gates (b) Pumps
   (c) Specific receptors (d) All of them
4. **The lipid composition of membranes are:**
   (a) Phospholipids (b) Glycolipids
   (c) Sterol-cholesterol (d) All of them
5. **The commonest phospholipid:**
   (a) Phosphoglycerides (b) Sphingomyelins
   (c) Both (a) and (b) (d) None of them
6. **The glycolipids are:**
   (a) Cerebroside (b) Ganglioside
   (c) Both (a) and (b) (d) None of them

7. **Ganglioside contains a branched chain of:**
   (a) Seven glucose (b) Single glucose
   (c) Seven galactose (d) Either (a) or (c)

8. **Cholesterol is found in:**
   (a) Mitochondria (b) Golgi complex
   (c) Nuclear membrane (d) All of them

9. **The major lipids in membranes contain:**
   (a) Hydrophobic region (b) Hydrophilic region
   (c) Both (a) and (b) (d) None of them

10. **The integral proteins are:**
    (a) Globular in shape (b) Amphipathic
    (c) Both (a) and (b) (d) None of them

11. **The integration of proteins into membrane can be explained by the hypothesis:**
    (a) Signal (b) Membrane trigger
    (c) Both (a) and (b) (d) None of them

12. **Gap junction mediate and regulate the passage of:**
    (a) Ions (b) Small molecules
    (c) Both (a) and (b) (d) None of them

13. **Connexions consist of proteins sub-unit in number:**
    (a) 6 (b) 8
    (c) 10 (d) 12

14. **Ion channels are:**
    (a) Proteins (b) Fats
    (c) Carbohydrates (d) Vitamins

15. **Aquaporin- AQP_1 is a:**
    (a) Homotetrametric glycoprotein
    (b) Heterotetrametric glycoprotein
    (c) Both (a) and (b)
    (d) None of them

16. **Extracellular matrix is composed of:**
    (a) Heteropolysaccharide (b) Fibrous proteins
    (c) Both (a) and (b) (d) None of them

17. Caveolae occurs mainly in:

(a) Muscles (b) Bones

(c) Blood (d) All of them

18. Above the transition temperature highly mobile lipids are in:

(a) Liquid crystal state (b) Solid state

(c) Gaseous state (d) None of them

19. Membrane proteins:

(a) Catalyse chemical reactions (b) Mediate flow of nutrients

(c) Both (a) and (b) (d) None of them

20. Transition temperature of biological membrane is in the range of:

(a) 10-20°C (b) 10-30°C

(c) 10-40°C (d) 10-50°C

21. Ionophores are organic molecules of:

(a) Bacterial origin (b) Viral origin

(c) Parasitic origin (d) None of them

22. Cytochrome C is:

(a) Lipid linked protein

(b) Peripheral membrane protein

(c) Integral membrane protein

(d) None of them

23. Inner mitochondrial membrane is permeable to:

(a) H^+ (b) OH^-

(c) K^+ (d) All of them

24. Due to the mobilities of lipids, lipids bilayer can be considered to be a:

(a) One dimensional protein (b) Two dimensional protein

(c) Both (a) and (b) (d) None of them

25. Chloride bicarbonate exchanger also known as:

(a) Anion exchange protein (b) Cation exchange protein

(c) Both (a) and (b) (d) None of them

26. Plasma membranes are involved in:

(a) Active transport (b) Facilitated diffusion

(c) Nerve impulse (d) All of them

27. Facilitated diffusion and active transport show specificity for:

(a) Ions (b) Sugars

(c) Amino acids (d) All of them

28. Transport system is described on the basis of function according to the:

(a) Number of molecules moved (b) Direction of movement

(c) Both (a) and (b) (d) None of them

29. In Antiport system, two molecules move in opposite direction:

(a) Na^+ in (b) Ca^{2+}out

(c) Both (a) and (b) (d) None of them

30. Myelin membrane is composed of:

(a) Glycosphingolipids (b) Cholesterol

(c) Proteins (d) All of them

31. Multiple sclerosis and Guillain Barre syndrome is caused by:

(a) Demyelination (b) Impaired nerve conduction

(c) Both (a) and (b) (d) None of them

32. Proteins in the membranes are classified as:

(a) Receptors (b) Transporters

(c) Enzymes (d) All of them

33. Membrane function can be affected by excess of:

(a) Cholesterol (b) Lysophospholipid

(c) Glycosphingolipids (d) All of them

34. Lipids aggregate and form:

(a) Micelle (b) Bilayers

(c) Both (a) and (b) (d) None of them

35. The lipids bilayers are ~ 60 Å thick as measured by:

(a) Electron microscopy (b) X-ray diffraction

(c) Both (a) and (b) (d) None of them

36. The lipid bilayer is thicker in:

(a) Gel state (b) Liquid crystal state

(c) Either (a) or (b) (d) Neither (a) or (b)

37. The transition temperature of a bilayer increases with:

(a) Chain length
(b) Degree of saturation
(c) Both (a) and (b)
(d) None of them

38. The fatty acids composition of their membrane lipids with ambient temperature can be modified by:

(a) Bacteria
(b) Cold blooded animals
(c) Both (a) and (b)
(d) None of them

39. Lipid rich myelinated membranes have a protein to lipid ratio of:

(a) 0.23
(b) 3.2
(c) 0.29
(d) 0.20

40. Protein rich inner membrane of mitochondria has a protein to lipid ratio of:

(a) 0.56
(b) 0.23
(c) 3.2
(d) 0.20

41. Lipids linked proteins are:

(a) Pre-nylated
(b) Fatty acylated
(c) Glycosylphosphatidyl inositol linked
(d) All of them

42. In fatty acylated proteins, membrane proteins are linked to:

(a) Myristic acid
(b) Palmitic acid
(c) Both (a) and (b)
(d) None of them

43. At physiological pH cytochrome C is:

(a) Anionic
(b) Cationic
(c) Neutral
(d) All of them

44. Biological membranes have:

(a) Similar properties
(b) Dis-similar properties
(c) Both (a) and (b)
(d) None of them

45. Membrane proteins vary in their lateral diffusion rates:

(a) 30-90% freely mobile
(b) Some immobile
(c) Some diffuse more slowly
(d) All of them

46. Caveolae occurring on muscle and epithelial cells participate in:

(a) Endocytosis
(b) Inter-cellular signaling
(c) Both (a) and (b)
(d) None of them

47. Lung surfactant contains % by weight:

(a) Phsophatidyl choline 70-80%
(b) Phospholipid 80-90%
(c) Both (a) and (b)
(d) None of them

48. By alveolar cells, lung surfactant is continuously:

(a) Synthesized
(b) Secreted
(c) Recycled
(d) All of them

49. A defect of spectrin synthesis causes hereditary spherocytosis in which erythrocytes are:

(a) Spheroidal
(b) Fragile
(c) Inflexible
(d) All of them

50. In hereditary spherocytosis, individual suffers from anemia due to:

(a) Erythrocyte lysis
(b) Removal of spherocytic cells
(c) Both (a) and (b)
(d) None of them

51. The enzymes synthesizing membrane lipids are mostly integral membrane proteins of endoplasmic reticulum only in:

(a) Eukaryotes
(b) Prokaryotes
(c) Both (a) and (b)
(d) None of them

52. Lipids synthesized by integral membrane proteins in plasma membrane only in:

(a) Eukaryotes
(b) Prokaryotes
(c) Both (a) and (b)
(d) None of them

53. On the two sides of biological membrane, equal proportion of lipid and protein components:

(a) Occurs
(b) Do not occur
(c) Both (a) and (b)
(d) None of them

54. Lipids in biological membrane are distributed:

(a) Symmetrically
(b) Asymmetrically
(c) Both (a) and (b)
(d) None of them

55. The lipids and proteins composition in apical and basolateral domain is:

(a) Different
(b) Same
(c) Slightly different
(d) None of them

56. Several viruses localize to lipid rafts:

(a) Influenza (b) Ebola

(c) Measels (d) All of them

57. Carrier ionophores increase the permeabilities of membrane to their selected ion by:

(a) Binding it

(b) Diffusing through membrane

(c) Releasing the ion on the other side

(d) All of them

58. Valinomycin containing D- and L- amino acid residue participates in:

(a) Ester linkage (b) Peptide linkage

(c) Both (a) and (b) (d) None of them

59. Aquaporins (mammalian) identified are expressed at high level in tissues:

(a) Kidney (b) Salivary glands

(c) Lacrimal glands (d) All of them

60. Aquaporins permit the passage of water molecules at:

(a) Extremely high rate (b) Low rate

(c) Extremely low rate (d) None of them

61. In lipid bilayer, globular proteins are embedded in:

(a) Regular way (b) Irregular way

(c) Remains as such (d) None of them

62. Intake of macromolecules by cells is:

(a) Endocytosis (b) Exocytosis

(c) Either (a) or (b) (d) None of them

63. Release of macromolecules by the cells to the outside is:

(a) Exocytosis (b) Endocytosis

(c) Either (a) or (b) (d) Neither (a) or (b)

64. Via exocytosis, the secretion of hormone occurs:

(a) Insulin (b) Parathyroid

(c) Both (a) and (b) (d) None of them

65. A good example of endocytosis is uptake of:

(a) Low density lipoprotein (b) High density lipoprotein

(c) Very low density lipoprotein (d) None of them

66. Specific carrier proteins have been isolated and characterized for the transport of:

(a) Glucose (b) Galactose

(c) Leucine (d) All of them

67. For the survival of cells, there should be:

(a) High K^+ concentration (b) Low Na^+ concentration

(c) Both (a) and (b) (d) None of them

68. For the transmission of nerve impulse, there is a need for:

(a) Na^+ gradients

(b) K^+ gradient across the plasma membrane

(c) Both (a) and (b)

(d) None of them

69. The enzyme Na^+ - K^+ ATPase consists of:

(a) 2 α - subunits (b) 2 β - subunits

(c) Both (a) and (b) (d) None of them

70. Insulin increases glucose transport in:

(a) Muscle (b) Adipose tissue

(c) Both (a) and (b) (d) None of them

Answer Key

1	(d)	19	(c)	37	(c)	55	(a)
2	(d)	20	(c)	38	(c)	56	(d)
3	(d)	21	(a)	39	(a)	57	(d)
4	(d)	22	(a)	40	(c)	58	(c)
5	(a)	23	(d)	41	(d)	59	(d)
6	(c)	24	(b)	42	(c)	60	(a)
7	(d)	25	(a)	43	(b)	61	(b)
8	(d)	26	(d)	44	(a)	62	(a)
9	(c)	27	(d)	45	(d)	63	(a)
10	(c)	28	(c)	46	(c)	64	(c)
11	(c)	29	(c)	47	(c)	65	(a)
12	(c)	30	(d)	48	(d)	66	(d)
13	(a)	31	(c)	49	(d)	67	(c)
14	(a)	32	(d)	50	(c)	68	(c)
15	(a)	33	(d)	51	(a)	69	(c)
16	(c)	34	(a)	52	(b)	70	(c)
17	(c)	35	(c)	53	(b)		
18	(a)	36	(d)	54	(b)		

Chapter 15

Cancer, Oncogens and Growth Factors

1. **Many cancers are associated with the abnormal production of:**
   (a) Carbohydrates (b) Fats
   (c) Proteins (d) Minerals
2. **The tumor markers are:**
   (a) Enzymes (b) Proteins
   (c) Hormones (d) All of them
3. **Cancer is caused by the groups:**
   (a) Radiant energy (b) Chemical compounds
   (c) Viruses (d) All of them
4. **DNA of gene is damaged by:**
   (a) Ultraviolet rays (b) X-rays
   (c) γ-rays (d) All of them
5. **Ultraviolet radiation may cause the formation of:**
   (a) Purine dimers (b) Pyrimidine dimers
   (c) Nucleoside dimers (d) Nucleotide dimers

6. **Carcinogenecity with radiant energy is to cause damage to:**
   (a) DNA (b) RNA
   (c) mRNA (d) tRNA

7. **Chemicals can cause human cancers upto:**
   (a) 60 per cent (b) 70 per cent
   (c) 80 per cent (d) 90 per cent

8. **The carcinogenic substances may be:**
   (a) Organic molecules (b) Inorganic molecules
   (c) Both (a) and (b) (d) None of them

9. **The ultimate carcinogen attacks nucleophilic group in:**
   (a) DNA (b) RNA
   (c) Protein (d) All of them

10. **The specific mono-oxygenase responsible for the metabolism of polycyclic aromatic hydrocarbons is termed as:**
    (a) Cytochrome P-448 (b) Cytochrome P-450
    (c) Cytochrome b (d) Cytochrome C

11. **Promoters can cause:**
    (a) Promotion (b) Initiation
    (c) Acceleration (d) Demotion

12. **The premier target in carcinogenesis is:**
    (a) DNA (b) RNA
    (c) rRNA (d) None of them

13. **Many tumor cells exhibit abnormal:**
    (a) Golgi bodies (b) RNA
    (c) Chromosomes (d) All of them

14. **Burkitt's lymphoma is a fast growing cancer caused by:**
    (a) Monocytes (b) β-lymphocytes
    (c) Neutrophils (d) Eosinophils

15. **Oncogenic viruses contain as their genome:**
    (a) DNA (b) RNA
    (c) Either of the two (d) Neither of the two

16. The tumor marker calcitonin is used in:
(a) Medullary carcinoma (b) Cancer of liver
(c) Either of the two (d) Neither of the two

17. Alpha-fetoprotein is used in:
(a) Cancer of liver (b) Medullary carcinoma
(c) Either of the two (d) Neither of the two

18. In all types of cancer, single tumor marker is:
(a) used (b) Not used
(c) Either of the two (d) Neither of the two

19. Tumor markers are detected in:
(a) Advanced stage (b) Early stage
(c) Either of the two (d) Neither of the two

20. In myeloma, mephalan alkylates:
(a) DNA (b) Other molecules
(c) Both (a) and (b) (d) None of them

21. Transversions are frequent in the cancer of:
(a) Lung (b) Liver
(c) Both (a) and (b) (d) None of them

22. In different cancers mutational spectrum:
(a) Differ (b) Does not differ
(c) Remains same (d) None of them

23. Mono-oxygenases and transferases cause the metabolism of:
(a) Procarcinogens (b) Other xenobiotics
(c) Both (a) and (b) (d) None of them

24. Cancer cells which exhibit multidrug resistance (MDR) have the amount of proteins:
(a) Increased (b) Decreased
(c) Remains same (d) None of them

25. Carcinoma-malignant tumor arise from:
(a) Epithelial tissues (b) Connective tissues
(c) Either of the two (d) Neither of the two

26. 80% cancers are caused by:

(a) Diet (b) Life style

(c) Use of therapeutic drugs (d) All of them

27. Breast cancer is caused by:

(a) Diethyl stilbestrol (b) Triphenylene ethylene

(c) Both (a) and (b) (d) None of them

28. The rate of oxygen consumption of cancer cells is:

(a) Below to that of normal cells (b) Above to that of normal cells

(c) Remains same (d) None of them

29. For the treatment of cancer, most effective compounds are:

(a) Mephalan (b) Cyclophosphamide

(c) Both (a) and (b) (d) None of them

30. Bulsulphan has a greater effect on:

(a) Granulopoiesis (b) Mylogenous leukemia

(c) Both (a) and (b) (d) None of them

31. Cancerous cells are characterized by:

(a) Unrestricted growth (b) Invasion on local tissues

(c) Both (a) and (b) (d) None of them

32. Organic carcinogens are:

(a) Methylcholanthrene (b) 2-naphthylamine

(c) Benzpyrene (d) All of them

33. Malignant tissue is more deficient in:

(a) Cytochrome C (b) Cytochrome oxidase

(c) Cytochrome a (d) None of them

34. In the development of cancer regulatory genes involved are:

(a) Oncogenes (b) Anti oncogenes

(c) Both (a) and (b) (d) None of them

35. Increased level of alpha-fetoprotein (AFP) in serum indicates the cancer of:

(a) Liver (b) Germ cells of testes

(c) Lungs (d) All of them

36. Elevated levels of AFP are observed in:

(a) Cirrhosis (b) Hepatitis
(c) Pregnancy (d) All of them

37. Measurement of serum AFP provides a sensitive index for:

(a) Tumor therapy (b) Detection of recurrence
(c) Both (a) and (b) (d) None of them

38. Cancer cells:

(a) Form multilayers (b) Can move freely
(c) Both (a) and (b) (d) None of them

39. Normal cells:

(a) Form monolayers (b) Cannot move freely
(c) Both (a) and (b) (d) None of them

40. The tumor cells:

(a) Have altered permeability
(b) Transport across membranes
(c) Both (a) and (b)
(d) None of them

41. In cancer cells, there is an increase in the synthesis of:

(a) DNA (b) RNA
(c) Both (a) and (b) (d) None of them

42. In tumor cells, there is an elevation in:

(a) Aerobic glycolysis (b) Anaerobic glycolysis
(c) Both (a) and (b) (d) None of them

43. In tumor cells, the degradation of pyrimidines is:

(a) Reduced (b) Elevated
(c) Remains same (d) None of them

44. In tumor cells, the production of growth factors is:

(a) Increased (b) Decreased
(c) Remains same (d) None of them

45. In cancer cells, there is a change in the structure of:

(a) Glycoproteins (b) Glycolipids
(c) Both (a) and (b) (d) None of them

46. Metastasis is the major cause of cancer related:

(a) Morbidity (b) Mortality

(c) Both (a) and (b) (d) None of them

47. Malignant tumors have high level of:

(a) Glycolytic enzymes (b) Phosphate

(c) Nicotinamide adenine dinucleotide (d) All of them

48. In most of the cancers, activity of enzymes of nucleic acid metabolism is:

(a) High (b) Low

(c) Remains same (d) None of them

49. Inhibitors of nucleic acid biosynthesis are responsible for establishing interdependence of:

(a) DNA synthesis (b) RNA synthesis

(c) Protein synthesis (d) All of them

50. Mitomycins are a group of:

(a) Bactericidal antibiotics (b) Cytotoxic antibiotics

(c) Both (a) and (b) (d) None of them

51. Stem cell therapy is applied to:

(a) Many types of cancers (b) Neurologic diseases

(c) Both (a) and (b) (d) None of them

52. Cancer and birth defects are due to:

(a) Abnormal cell division (b) Abnormal differentiation

(c) Both (a) and (b) (d) None of them

53. Disturbances in the transcription are involved in:

(a) Heart disease (b) Cancer

(c) Various kinds of inflammation (d) All of them

54. Transcriptional regulation underlies the aspects of cellular metabolism:

(a) Morphogenesis (Development) (b) Oncogenesis (cancer)

(c) Both (a) and (b) (d) None of them

55. Apoptosis acts as a biological link between:

(a) Cancer genetics (b) Cancer therapy

(c) Both (a) and (b) (d) None of them

56. The development of malignant tumour cells results from:
(a) Deregulated proliferation
(b) Inability of cells to undergo death
(c) Either (a) or (b)
(d) Neither (a) or (b)

57. Disregulation of apoptosis results in:
(a) Cancer (b) Auto immune disorder
(c) Ischemic injuries (d) All of them

58. There is remarkable increase in cell death, where the apoptosis is disabled by:
(a) Dominant oncogens
(b) Agents disrupting anti-apoptic function
(c) Both (a) and (b)
(d) None of them

59. Massive cell death can occur, where the apoptosis is lost:
(a) Restoring dysfunctional gene (b) By a mutation
(c) Restoring the activity (d) All of them

60. Since apoptic pathway can be manipulated to produce massive changes in cell death, the drug targets are:
(a) Genes (b) Proteins
(c) Both (a) and (b) (d) None of them

Answer Key

1	(c)	16	(a)	31	(c)	46	(c)
2	(d)	17	(a)	32	(d)	47	(d)
3	(d)	18	(b)	33	(a)	48	(a)
4	(d)	19	(a)	34	(c)	49	(d)
5	(b)	20	(c)	35	(d)	50	(c)
6	(a)	21	(c)	36	(d)	51	(c)
7	(c)	22	(a)	37	(c)	52	(c)
8	(c)	23	(c)	38	(c)	53	(d)
9	(d)	24	(a)	39	(c)	54	(c)
10	(a)	25	(a)	40	(c)	55	(c)
11	(b)	26	(d)	41	(c)	56	(c)
12	(a)	27	(c)	42	(c)	57	(d)
13	(c)	28	(a)	43	(a)	58	(c)
14	(b)	29	(c)	44	(a)	59	(d)
15	(c)	30	(c)	45	(c)	60	(c)

Chapter 16

Clinical Biochemistry

1. **Hyperventillation will lead to:**
   (a) Metabolic acidosis (b) Metabolic alkalosis
   (c) Respiratory acidosis (d) Respiratory alkalosis
2. **Acute diarrhoea in a young calf can lead to:**
   (a) Metabolic acidosis (b) Hyperkalemia
   (c) Hyperglycemia (d) All of them
3. **Steatorrhoea is seen in:**
   (a) Diarrhoea (b) Vomiting
   (c) Intestinal malabsorption (d) All of them
4. **Which of the following is not a ketone body?**
   (a) Aceto acetate (b) β-hydroxy butyrate
   (c) Oxaloacetate (d) Acetone
5. **Increased levels of which of the following is indicative of hepatopathy?**
   (a) Lipase (b) Creatine kinase
   (c) Arginase (d) All of them
6. **Ketonuria may be observed in:**
   (a) Bovine ketosis (b) Ovine pregnancy toxemia
   (c) Prolonged starvation (d) All of them

7. **Which of the following is not a function of ruminant saliva?**
   (a) Urea recycling
   (b) Buffering
   (c) Lubrication
   (d) Carbohydrate digestion

8. **The normal osmolality of plasma is:**
   (a) 285-295 milliosmoles/kg
   (b) 295-395 milliosmoles/kg
   (c) 395-495 milliosmoles/kg
   (d) None of them

9. **The body acid load is predominantly eliminated in the form of:**
   (a) NH_4^+
   (b) Na^+
   (c) Both (a) and (b)
   (d) None of them

10. **Most of the biotransformation reactions occur in:**
    (a) Intestine
    (b) Liver
    (c) Kidney
    (d) Brain

11. **Which of the following is most likely to induce a strong immune response?**
    (a) Phospholipid
    (b) Glycolipid
    (c) Glycoprotein
    (d) Polynucleotide

12. **Ancestral antibody is:**
    (a) IgA
    (b) IgD
    (c) IgE
    (d) IgM

13. **Severe vomiting can result in:**
    (a) Hyponatremia
    (b) Hypokalemia
    (c) Hyperchloremia
    (d) Hyperkalemia

14. **Decreased CSF glucose reflects:**
    (a) Acute meningitis
    (b) Bacterial meningitis
    (c) Fungal meningitis
    (d) All of them

15. **Which of the following is a liver specific enzyme?**
    (a) Acid phosphatase
    (b) Creatine kinase
    (c) Alanine aminotransferase
    (d) Amylase

16. **Which of the following contributes to buffering by hemoglobin?**
    (a) Lysine
    (b) Histidine
    (c) Leucine
    (d) Arginine

17. Hyperglycemia can be observed in:

(a) Encephalitis
(b) Meningitis
(c) Hyperadrenocorticism
(d) All of them

18. BUN level rises in:

(a) Hepatic failure
(b) Kidney failure
(c) Biliary obstruction
(d) Pancreatic insufficiency

19. The primary defect in metabolic acidosis is a reduction in the plasma concentration of:

(a) Bicarbonate
(b) Carbonic acid
(c) Both (a) and (b)
(d) None of them

20. Carboxyhemoglobin is formed by:

(a) CO
(b) CO_2
(c) HCO_3
(d) HCN

21. The most abundantly available base in plasma is:

(a) Na^+
(b) K^+
(c) Ca^+
(d) All of them

22. Which of the following is not a phase II reaction of xenobiotic metabolism?

(a) Hydroxylation
(b) Glucuronidation
(c) Sulfation
(d) Acetylation

23. Spontaneous decarboxylation of acetoacetate in hepatic cells will result in the formation of:

(a) Acetaldehyde
(b) Acetyl CoA
(c) Acetone
(d) Acetic acid

24. CNS depressants usage may cause one of the following conditions:

(a) Respiratory acidosis
(b) Respiratory alkalosis
(c) Metabolic acidosis
(d) Metabolic alkalosis

25. Inulin clearance test is used for the detection of function of:

(a) Liver
(b) Lungs
(c) Pancreas
(d) Kidney

26. Deficiency of de-branching enzyme leading to accumulation of abnormal glycogen is:

(a) Pompe's disease
(b) Cori's disease
(c) Anderson's disease
(d) Van Gierke's disease

27. One of the following species of animals do not suffer from diabetes:

(a) Dogs (b) Cattle

(c) Cats (d) Rats

28. Enzyme isocitrate dehydrogenase level in serum will increase in:

(a) Cirrhosis (b) Diabetes mellitus

(c) Brain tumor (d) Lung cancer

29. BMR test is done to assess the activity of:

(a) Adrenaline (b) Oestrogen

(c) Thyroxine (d) Insulin

30. Choline fraction of phospholipids when degraded by intestinal bacteria will yield a toxin called:

(a) Histamine (b) Putricine

(c) Neurine (d) Cadavarine

31. The immunoglobulin not having antibody activity:

(a) IgE (b) IgM

(c) IgG (d) IgD

32. Major non protein nitrogenous substance found in urine of animals is:

(a) Uric acid (b) Creatinine

(c) Urea (d) Hypoxanthine

33. The number of molecules of oxygen taken by hemoglobin is:

(a) 1 (b) 2

(c) 3 (d) 4

34. The probable metabolic defect in gout is:

(a) An overproduction of calcium

(b) An overproduction of pyrimidine

(c) An overproduction of uric acid

(d) Rise in calcium leading to calcium urate deposition

35. In ruminants which ketone body is increased in blood:

(a) Aceto acetic acid (b) β-hydroxybutyric acid

(c) Propanol (d) All of them

36. An increase in blood urea/uremia in animals occurs in:

(a) Severe and prolonged vomiting and diarrhoea

(b) Haemorrhage and shock

(c) Ulcers and stones in urinary tract

(d) All of them

37. Burkitt's is a fast growing tumor of:

(a) Monocytes (b) B-lymphocytes

(c) Neutrophils (d) Eosinophils

38. The specific mono-oxygenase responsible for metabolism of polycyclic aromatic hydrocarbon is:

(a) Cytochrome P-448 (b) Cytochrome P-450

(c) Cytochrome b (d) None of them

39. Bohr effect shifts the oxygen dissociation curve:

(a) From right to left (b) From left to right

(c) Either left or right (d) None of them

40. Oxygen is supplied to the tissues in the form of:

(a) Simple physical solution (b) Oxyhemoglobin

(c) Both (a) and (b) (d) None of them

41. Major proportion of CO_2 is transported as:

(a) Physically dissolved CO_2 (b) Carbaminohemoglobin

(c) Bicarbonate (d) Carboxyhemoglobin

42. Chief antibody of the secondary immune response is:

(a) IgG (b) IgM

(c) IgE (d) IgD

43. The precursor for steroid biosynthesis is:

(a) Tyrosine (b) VFA

(c) Cholesterol (d) None of them

44. Impairment in the synthesis of dopamine by the brain is a major causative factor for the disorder:

(a) Parkinson's disease (b) Addison's disease

(c) Cushing syndrome (d) Goiter

45. The normal ratio of carbonic acid to bicarbonate is:

(a) 1:20
(b) 1:15
(c) 1:18
(d) 1:10

46. The transport of glucose across the cell membrane is facilitated by:

(a) Glucagon
(b) Insulin
(c) Thyroxine
(d) Gonadotropin

47. Bile stones are formed in liver and gall bladder when bile acid: cholesterol ratio:

(a) Falls below critical value
(b) Increases above critical value
(c) Both (a) and (b)
(d) None of them

48. When the amount of hemoglobin in the body is reduced below the normal, the hypoxia is termed as:

(a) Hypoxic hypoxia
(b) Anemic hypoxia
(c) Stagnant hypoxia
(d) Histonic hypoxia

49. The no. of iron atoms in ferrous state per mole of hemoglobin:

(a) 1
(b) 2
(c) 3
(d) 4

50. Carbon dioxide in blood is transported as:

(a) Physical solution
(b) Carbonic acid
(c) Bicarbonate
(d) All of them

51. Steatorrhoea is prominent in blood as:

(a) Acute diarrhoea
(b) Volvulus
(c) Ischemia
(d) Intestinal malabsorption

52. The major class of immunoglobulin present in colostrum of ruminants is:

(a) IgE
(b) IgD
(c) IgA
(d) IgM

53. Serum amylase activity is significantly increased in:

(a) Pancreatitis
(b) Obstructive jaundice
(c) Prostatic carcinoma
(d) Hepatic cell necrosis

54. The metabolic water is derived by the oxidation of:

(a) Carbohydrates (b) Proteins

(c) Fats (d) All of them

55. The most predominant anion in the extracellular fluid is:

(a) Cl^- (b) HCO_3^-

(c) HPO_4^{2-} (d) None of them

56. The only route through which H^+ are eliminated from the body:

(a) Lungs (b) Stomach

(c) Kidney (d) None of them

57. Respiratory alkalosis is primarily associated with decrease in plasma concentration is:

(a) Carbonic acid (b) Bicarbonate

(c) Both (a) and (b) (d) None of them

58. Na^+ reabsorption by renal tubules is increased by hormone:

(a) Aldosterone (b) Testosterone

(c) Both (a) and (b) (d) None of them

59. Oxidation occurs mainly in:

(a) Liver (b) Kidney

(c) Intestine (d) All of them

60. Glycine is the conjugating agent for:

(a) Alcohols (b) Phenols

(c) Amines (d) Carboxylic acid

61. Sulphur of organic compounds may be excreted as:

(a) Organic sulphates (b) Inorganic sulphates

(c) Neutral sulphur (d) All of them

62. The anion gap refers to the unmeasured plasma anion concentration (in the laboratory) and is represented by:

(a) Proteins and organic acids (b) Phosphates and sulphates

(c) Urates (d) All of them

63. Name the amino acid from which ammonia is derived in the renal tubular cells which is finally excreted as NH_4^+:

(a) Asparagine (b) Glutamine

(c) Glutamate (d) Aspartate

64. Oxidation and conjugation occur exclusively in:

(a) Lungs
(b) Heart
(c) Liver
(d) All of them

65. Which of the following has important role in maintenance of ECV?

(a) ADH
(b) Rennin-Angiotensin
(c) ANF
(d) Cortisol

66. Chronic vomiting results in:

(a) Hyper chloremia
(b) Hypophosphatemia
(c) Hypokalemia
(d) All of them

67. Many toxins are:

(a) Hepatotoxic
(b) Nephrotoxic
(c) Both (a) and (b)
(d) None of them

68. Which of the following results in acute diarrhoea?

(a) Hypermotility
(b) Maldigestion
(c) Hypersecretion of water and electrolytes
(d) All of them

69. Which of the following is observed in acute vomition?

(a) Metabolic acidosis
(b) Metabolic alkalosis
(c) Chronic acidosis
(d) Respiratory alkalosis

70. The source of energy in prolonged starvation for brain is:

(a) Only glucose
(b) Only ketone bodies
(c) Glucose and ketone bodies
(d) None of them

71. The long term compensatory response by kidney for metabolic acidosis are:

(a) Conservation of HCO_3^-
(b) Generation of HCO_3^-
(c) Secretion of H^+
(d) All of them

72. Which of the following is not a cause of metabolic acidosis?

(a) Ketosis
(b) Renal failure
(c) Diarrhoea
(d) Acute vomition

73. The detoxication reactions are mainly carried out in:

(a) Liver
(b) Heart
(c) Intestine
(d) None of them

74. In alkalosis urinary ammonia:

(a) Decreases
(b) Increases
(c) Remains same
(d) None of them

75. The amount of nitrogen in inspired air and expired air is:

(a) Same
(b) Higher
(c) Lower
(d) None of the above

76. Glucuronic acid is the conjugating agent for:

(a) Alcohols
(b) Phenols
(c) Carboxylic acid
(d) All of them

77. The best conjugating agent for amino compounds is:

(a) Glucuronic acid
(b) Glycine
(c) Acetic acid
(d) Sulphuric acid

78. Normal level of cholesterol in goat blood is:

(a) 10mg/100ml
(b) 90mg/100ml
(c) 300mg/100ml
(d) None of them

79. Ketone bodies consist of:

(a) Acetone
(b) Acetoacetic acid
(c) β-hydroxybutyric acid
(d) All of them

80. Normal value of creatine kinase is:

(a) 10-50 IU/L
(b) 5-25 IU/L
(c) 20-50 IU/L
(d) 0-10 IU/L

81. Normal value of AST is:

(a) 4-45 IU/L
(b) 4-20 IU/L
(c) 20-50 IU/L
(d) 0-10 IU/L

82. Renal threshold for glucose is:

(a) 160-180 mg/100ml
(b) 260-280mg/100ml
(c) 10-100mg/100ml
(d) 50-100mg/100ml

83. Clinical features of diabetes mellitus are:

(a) Marked loss of weight
(b) Appearance of sugar in urine
(c) Excretion of large volume of urine
(d) All of them

84. The serum enzyme elevated in alcoholic cirrhosis of liver is:
(a) Alanine transaminase (b) Aspartate transaminase
(c) Alcohol dehydrogenase (d) γ-glutamyl transpeptidase

85. Name the immunoglobulin involved in body allergic reactions:
(a) IgA (b) IgE
(c) IgD (d) IgM

86. An adult man secrets on an average:
(a) 1-1.5 L saliva (b) 4-5 L saliva
(c) 2-8 L saliva (d) 10-20 L saliva

87. The pH value of pancreatic juice lies in the range of:
(a) 1.5-2.5 (b) 4.5-5.5
(c) 7.5-8.2 (d) 8.5-9.5

88. The amount of bile secreted by liver daily is:
(a) 200-600ml (b) 500-1000ml
(c) 700-1500ml (d) 800-1800ml

89. BAL is used as detoxicating agent for the removal of:
(a) Lewisite (b) Toxic metals
(c) Both (a) and (b) (d) None of them

90. Cyanides are detoxified in the body by:
(a) Methylation (b) Reaction with thiosulphate
(c) Reaction with cysteine (d) Reaction with acetic acid

91. Glycine is the conjugating agent for:
(a) Alcohol (b) Phenol
(c) Amines (d) Carboxylic acid

92. Which one is the natural anticoagulant?
(a) Sodium oxalate (b) Potassium oxalate
(c) Heparin (d) Ammonium oxalate

93. Foreign bodies entering the body are:
(a) Antibodies (b) Antigens
(c) Antibiotics (d) Immunoglobulins

94. The amount of oxygen (Volume per cent) is maximum in:

(a) Inspired air (b) Expired air

(c) Alveolar air (d) All of them

95. Oxyhemoglobin can transport:

(a) 2ml CO_2/100ml blood (b) 3ml CO_2/100ml blood

(c) 5ml CO_2/100ml blood (d) 8ml CO_2/100ml blood

96. Hepatic injury caused by toxin is due to the role of liver in:

(a) Biotransformation (b) Disposition of xenobiotics

(c) Both (a) and (b) (d) None of them

97. The serum enzyme used to evaluate pancreatic function:

(a) Alkaline phosphatase (b) Amylase

(c) Lactate dehydrogenase (d) Acid phosphatase

98. Aromatic hydrocarbons are oxidized to:

(a) Phenols (b) Acids

(c) Amines (d) None of them

99. Chief antibody of secondary immune response is:

(a) IgG (b) IgM

(c) IgE (d) IgD

100. Which of the following immunoglobulin in a penta polymer each consisting of two light and two heavy chains?

(a) IgG (b) IgM

(c) IgA (d) IgE

101. The hormones that differ least in chemical structure are:

(a) Insulin and pro-insulin

(b) Oxytocin and vasopressin

(c) Cortisone and growth stimulating hormone

(d) Thyrotropin and oxytocin

102. The gene for synthesis of insulin is located on chromosome:

(a) 9 (b) 11

(c) 13 (d) 15

103. The blood pH is normally maintained at:

(a) 7.0 (b) 7.4

(c) 7.8 (d) 7.6

104. The oxygen dissociation curve of hemoglobin is:

(a) Sigmoidal (b) Hyperbolic

(c) Semilunar (d) Circular

105. Benzoic acid in conjugation with glycine yields:

(a) Hippuric acid (b) Uric acid

(c) Histidine (d) Urea

106. The flexible region of immunoglobulin structure is:

(a) Fab (b) Fc

(c) Hinge region (d) J-chain

107. An acute blood loss leads to:

(a) Neurogenic shock (b) Hypovoluemic shock

(c) Thermal shock (d) Metabolic shock

108. Majority of CO_2 produced from tissue is transported to lungs as:

(a) Bicarbonate (b) Carbonic acid

(c) Carbamino Hb (d) Oxy Hb

109. Name of hormone predominantly produced in flight, fright and fight:

(a) Thyroxine (b) Aldosterone

(c) Epinephrine (d) ADH

110. SGOT increases in:

(a) Heart attack (b) Ricket

(c) Muscular dystrophy (d) None of them

111. Nephrotoxic antibiotics are:

(a) Amino glycosides (b) Sulfonamides

(c) Tetracyclines (d) All of them

112. The urinary excretion of ketoacids derived from branched chain amino acids produces an odour like that of:

(a) Maple syrup (b) Burnt sugar

(c) Either (a) or (b) (d) Neither (a) or (b)

113. The effect of CO_2 on oxygen carrying capacity of hemoglobin is known is:

(a) Bohr effect (b) Pasteur effect

(c) Tension effect (d) Hamburger effect

114. Serum uric acid is increased in:

(a) Gout (b) Rheumatoid arthritis
(c) Leukemia (d) All of them

115. The normal adult level of total bilirubin in plasma is:

(a) 0 to 1.5mg/100ml (b) 0.6 to 0.9mg/100ml
(c) 0.1 to 1.2mg/100ml (d) 0.4 to 0.8mg/100ml

116. Elevated SGPT level is seen in:

(a) Hepatitis (b) Acute pancreatitis
(c) Alcoholism (d) None of the above

117. Acid phosphatase increases in:

(a) Cancer of prostrate gland (b) Liver disease
(c) Heart attack (d) Muscular dystrophy

118. SGOT increases in:

(a) Heart attack (b) Ricket
(c) Muscular dystrophy (d) None of the above

119. Alkaline phosphatase increases in:

(a) Alcoholism (b) Myocardial infarction
(c) Acute pancreatitis (d) None of the above

120. Creatinine phosphokinase increases in:

(a) Myocardial infarction (b) Alcoholism
(c) Pancreatic dystrophy (d) None of the above

121. Aldolase increases in:

(a) Muscular dystrophy (b) Alcoholism
(c) Ricket (d) None of them

122. Normal value of acid phosphatase is:

(a) 2.5-12 IU/L (b) 1.0-2.0 IU/L
(c) 5.0-7.5 IU/L (d) 0.5-1.0 IU/L

123. Normal value of ALT is:

(a) 3-40 IU/L (b) 1-20 IU/L
(c) 0-10 IU/L (d) 2-10 IU/L

124. α-glutamyl transpeptidase activity in serum is elevated in:

(a) Pancreatitis
(b) Muscular dystrophy
(c) Myocardial infarction
(d) Alcoholism

125. Hyper cholestermia is observed in:

(a) Hypothyroidism
(b) Diabetes mellitus
(c) Nephrotic syndrome
(d) All of them

126. By decreasing the solubility of colloidal antigen, their antigenicity is usually:

(a) Increased
(b) Decreased
(c) Both (a) and (b)
(d) None of them

127. Higher the molecular weight, more is the:

(a) Antigenecity
(b) Immunogenecity
(c) Both (a) and (b)
(d) None of them

128. All immunological molecules on the surface of a given β-cells have the same:

(a) Isotype
(b) Idiotype
(c) Both (a) and (b)
(d) None of them

129 For hepatocellular injury in dog and cat following enzyme is nearly specific:

(a) ALT
(b) AST
(c) Both (a) and (b)
(d) None of them

130. Calves fed a milk diet that may lead to hypomagnesemia develop a decreased activity of:

(a) Thyroid
(b) Insulin
(c) Glucagon
(d) Epinephrine

131. Pleocytosis is:

(a) Increase in cellularity of CSF
(b) Decrease in cellularity of CSF
(c) Both (a) and (b)
(d) None of them

132. In the diagnosis of myocardial infarction, important enzymes are:

(a) CPK
(b) AST
(c) LDH
(d) All of them

133. In multiple myeloma increased production of immunoglobulin is observed:

(a) IgA (b) IgD
(c) IgE (d) Any one

134. Respiratory distress syndrome in infants is characterized by:

(a) Presence of dipalmitoyl lecithin
(b) Absence of dipalmitoyl lecithin
(c) Both (a) and (b)
(d) None of them

135. Genetic diseases impending protein maturation are:

(a) Scrapie (b) Alzheimer disease
(c) Mad cow disease (d) All of them

136. Immunoglobulin M accounts for:

(a) 5-10% (b) 10-20%
(c) 20-40% (d) 0-5%

137. Best antigens are:

(a) Lipids (b) Polysaccharides
(c) Proteins (d) Nucleic acids

138. The basic structure of an antibody is an unit consisting of:

(a) 6 (b) 9
(c) 5 (d) 4, polypeptide chains

139. An interaction between an antibody and an antigen depends on:

(a) 3 (b) 4
(c) 5 (d) 6, types of non-covalent forces

140. Ceruloplasmin is associated with:

(a) Wilson disease (b) Goitre
(c) Parkinson's disease (d) None of them

141. Disease caused by protein misfolding:

(a) Alzheimer disease
(b) Amyloidoses
(c) Transmiscible spongiform encephalopathies
(d) All of them

142. In proteinuria, urine contains:

(a) More plasma proteins (b) Enzymes
(c) Both (a) and (b) (d) None of them

143. In enzymuria, the followings are reflected:

(a) Renal diseases (b) Nephrotoxicosis
(c) Both (a) and (b) (d) None of them

144. An increase in serum unspecific alkaline phosphatase is an indication of cholestasis in:

(a) Dogs (b) Rats
(c) Man (d) All of them

145. In plasma, enzymes are elevated in:

(a) Cell damage (b) Enzyme induction
(c) Both (a) and (b) (d) All of them

146. AST found in:

(a) Cytosol (b) Mitochondria
(c) Both (a) and (b) (d) None of them

147. Respiratory distress syndrome is due to difficulty in:

(a) Mastication (b) Breathing
(c) Swallowing (d) Chewing

148. Fasting blood glucose level (mg/100ml) is:

(a) 90 (b) 120
(c) 160 (d) 180

149. McArdle's disease's clinical features are:

(a) Muscle cramps (b) Pain
(c) Weakness (d) All of them

150. Ovine pregnancy toxemia is associated with:

(a) Hypoglycemia (b) Ketonemia
(c) Ketonuria (d) All of them

151. Ketonemia in diabetes is due to:

(a) Increased Lipolysis
(b) Accelerated hepatic gluconeogenesis
(c) Both (a) and (b)
(d) None of them

152. Nephrotoxic metals include:

(a) Arsenic
(b) Cadmium
(c) Lead
(d) All of them

153. Clinical signs associated with lysosomal storage disorders are:

(a) Growth retardation
(b) Umbilical hernia
(c) Corneal clouding
(d) All of them

154. Clinical signs of uremia are:

(a) Cerebral dysfunction
(b) EEG alteration
(c) Peripheral neuropathy
(d) All of them

155. In normal CSF, eosinophils are:

(a) Present
(b) Absent
(c) Both (a) and (b)
(d) None of them

156. Toxins inducing hemolysis may produce:

(a) Anemia
(b) Icterus
(c) Hemoglobinuria
(d) All of them

157. Necrosis of skeletal muscles results in:

(a) Myoglobinemia
(b) Hyperkalemia
(c) Both (a) and (b)
(d) None of them

158. Glycogen storage disease II is caused by the deficiency of:

(a) Acid α-glucosidase
(b) β-galactosidase
(c) β-glucuronidase
(d) α-facosidase

159. In spontaneous ketosis, milk production is:

(a) Decreased
(b) Increased
(c) Remains same
(d) None of them

160. Sickle cell anemia is due to change in single nucleotide of:

(a) β-globulin gene
(b) α-globulin gene
(c) γ-globulin gene
(d) All of them

161. Porphyrins are cyclic compounds composed of pyrrole rings:

(a) 4
(b) 3
(c) 2
(d) 5

162. Diabetes mellitus caused by the deficiency in the secretion of:

(a) Insulin (b) Glucagon

(c) Both (a) and (b) (d) All of them

163. Atherosclerosis is correlated with increased:

(a) LDL (b) HDL

(c) VLDL (d) All of them

164. Anderson disease affects:

(a) Liver (b) Heart

(c) Muscle (d) All of them

165. Phenylketonuria is characterized by:

(a) Physical retardation (b) Pain in joints

(c) Nephrons (d) Mental retardation

166. In order to suppress immunologic rejection in organ transplantation is:

(a) Azathioprine (b) Allopurinol

(c) 5-Iododeoxyuridine (d) 6-azacytidine

167. In most instances, serum enzyme determinations are used as screening test to detect organ involvement, most desirable are:

(a) High sensitivity (b) Reasonable specificity

(c) Both (a) and (b) (d) None of them

168. Erythropenia is observed in:

(a) Phenothiazine toxicity (b) Brucellosis

(c) Diarrhoea (d) Vomiting

169. Hemoglobin level becomes low in:

(a) Polycythemia (b) Equine influenza

(c) Strangles (d) Dehydration

170. For brain tumor diagnosis, cells present in _____ may provide diagnosis:

(a) Synovial fluid (b) Serum

(c) Urine (d) CSF

171. Canine pellagra is caused by the deficiency of:

(a) Nicotinic acid (b) Pyridoxine

(c) Choline (d) Biotin

172. Hypervitaminosis A may cause:
(a) Osteopetrosis (b) Osteomalacia
(c) Osteoporosis (d) None of them

173. Hypophosphataemia causes:
(a) Pica (b) Rheumatism like syndrome
(c) Hemoglobinuria (d) All of them

174. Chronic selenium toxicity causes:
(a) Muscular dystrophy (b) Rickets
(c) Parakeratosis (d) Blind staggers

175. Steely wool is a characteristic symptom of:
(a) Iodine (b) Manganese
(c) Cobalt (d) Copper

176. Chronic respiratory disease is caused by:
(a) Mycoplasma (b) *E. coli*
(c) Both (a) and (b) (d) None of them

177. Decreased cholinesterase activity is observed in:
(a) Organ phosphate poisoning (b) Carbamate poisoning
(c) Both (a) and (b) (d) None of them

178. Mercury poisoning produces:
(a) Anuria (b) Ulcers in stomach
(c) Endocardial hemorrhage (d) All of them

179. Degnala disease is characterized by:
(a) Gangrene on tail (b) Pneumonia
(c) Enteritis (d) None of them

180. Aflatoxicosis causes _____ in poultry:
(a) Immunosuppresion (b) Drop in egg production
(c) Hepatitis (d) All of them

181. Azotemia is the clinical condition associated with:
(a) Reduced renal arterial tension
(b) Retention of nitrogen wastes in blood
(c) Both (a) and (b)
(d) None of them

182. Severe vomiting produces loss of large quantities of:

(a) Water
(b) H^+ ions
(c) Cl^- ions
(d) All of them

183. Vomiting does occurs in:

(a) Cat
(b) Dog
(c) Horse
(d) Pig

184. In gastric dilation volvulus the result is accumulation of:

(a) Gas
(b) Fluid in stomach
(c) Both (a) and (b)
(d) None of them

185. Distenion and displacement of stomach causes obstruction of:

(a) Caudal venacava
(b) Portal vein
(c) Both (a) and (b)
(d) None of them

186. Hypovolemic shock is the result of:

(a) Decrease in cardiac output
(b) Decrease in arterial blood pressure
(c) Tissue perfusion
(d) All of them

187. Hemoconcentration and increased TSP were attributed to fluid shifts from vascular compartment into the:

(a) Lumen of alimentary tract
(b) Wall of stomach
(c) Wall of peritoneal cavity
(d) All of them

188. The re-perfusion injury is caused in part by:

(a) Oxygen free radicals (OFR)
(b) Superoxide (O_2^-)
(c) Hydroxyl free radicals (OH^-)
(d) All of them

189. The re-perfusion injury is characterized by increased:

(a) Microvascular permeability
(b) Mucosal permeability
(c) Mucosal necrosis
(d) All of them

190. The formation of oxygen free radical is preceded by accumulation of:

(a) Hypoxanthine in endothelial cells
(b) Intestinal mucosal cells during ischemia
(c) Both (a) and (b)
(d) None of them

191. K^+ deficiency and hypovolemia caused by dehydration may result in:

(a) Renal tubular damage (b) Renal failure

(c) Both (a) and (b) (d) None of them

192. Via lipid peroxidation, hydroxyl free radicals (OH^-) initiate:

(a) Structural cellular membrane damage

(b) Functional cellular membrane damage

(c) Both (a) or (b)

(d) None of them

193. During lipid peroxidation neutrophils are recruited into ischemic and reperfused tissue by:

(a) Xanthine oxidase derived oxygen free radicals

(b) Chemoattractants released from cellular membrane

(c) Both (a) and (b)

(d) None of them

194. Increased cystosolic calcium concentration during ischemia and subsequent lipid peroxidation activate phospholipase which in turn causes the release of:

(a) Platelet activating factor

(b) Metabolites of arachidonic acid

(c) Metabolites of lysophosphatidyl choline

(d) All of them

195. Infiltration and degranulation in affected tissue is promoted by:

(a) Leukotriene B_4 (b) Thromboxane A_2

(c) Plate let activating factor (d) All of them

196. In the experimental and clinical studies of ischemic reperfusion injury, the pharmacological agents used are:

(a) Xanthine oxidase inhibitors (b) Deferroxamine

(c) Cyclo-oxygenase (d) All of them

197. In diarrhoea, decreased intestinal assimilation of nutrients that may result from maldigestion due to:

(a) Pancreatic exocrine insufficiency

(b) Bile salt deficiency

(c) Defective mucosal transport of cell

(d) Either (a), (b) or (c)

198. Acute diarrhoea represents the leading cause of morbidity and mortality in:

(a) Neonatal calves (b) Pigs

(c) Both (a) and (b) (d) None of them

199. Intestinal malabsorption is associated with intestinal disease like:

(a) Chronic inflammatory disease (b) Granulomatous disease

(c) Lymphoma (d) All of them

200. Clinical signs of intestinal malabsorption are:

(a) Persistent diarrhoea (b) Weight loss

(c) Steatorrhoea (d) All of them

201. Primary end products of rumen fermentation are:

(a) Short chain fatty acids (b) Long chain fatty acids

(c) Either (a) or (b) (d) Neither (a) or (b)

202. Abrupt change in the diet results in:

(a) Acute rumen indigestion (b) Acute rumen tympany

(c) Urea poisoning (d) All of them

203. Ruminants can meet their dietary protein requirement by the use of:

(a) Urea (b) Biuret

(c) Ammonium salts (d) All of them

204. Acute toxicity of skeletal/cardiac muscle can be detected by elevation in:

(a) Bilirubin (b) Serum creatine kinase

(c) Both (a) and (b) (d) None of them

205. In uremia, nervous system is affected:

(a) Centrally (b) Peripherally

(c) Both (a) and (b) (b) None of them

206. In uremia, the following is seen:

(a) Abnormalities in leucocytes number (b) Abnormality in platelet function

(c) Shortening of red cell survival time (d) All of them

207. Uremia causes suppression of immune system and impairs:

(a) Humoral factors (b) Cellular factors

(c) Both (a) and (b) (d) None of them

208. During uremia, drug oxidations by microsomal oxidative system are:

(a) Normal (b) Accelerated

(c) Either (a) or (b) (d) Neither (a) or (b)

209. In Uremia alteration in the metabolism seen of:

(a) Protein (b) Lipid

(c) Both (a) and (b) (d) None of them

210. In uremia:

(a) HDL level increased (b) VLDL increased

(c) Decrease in HDL (d) Both (b) and (c)

211. Cerebrospinal fluid is hazy/turbid due to:

(a) Micro-organisms (b) Epidural fat

(c) Myelographic contrast agent (d) (a) or (b) or (c)

212. The colour of cerebrospinal fluid (CSF) is:

(a) Yellow (b) Pink

(c) Brown (d) (a) or (b) or (c)

213. If the cerebrospinal fluid protein level is increased, colour change will be:

(a) Greater (b) Lesser

(c) Remains same (d) None of them

214. Viscosity of cerebrospinal fluid increases due to:

(a) Very high CSF protein content (b) Cryptococcosis

(c) Epidural fat (d) All of them

215. Cerebrospinal fluid eosinophilia can occur in association with the infection of type:

(a) Bacterial (b) Viral

(c) Fungal (d) All of them

216. Cerebrospinal fluid eosinophilia is caused by:

(a) Bacterial encephalitis (b) Neosporosis

(c) Toxoplasmosis (d) All of them

217. Increased total protein content of CSF may be caused by increased permeability of blood of:

(a) Brain (b) Spinal cord

(c) CSF barriers (d) (a) or (b) or (c)

218. Low CSF protein is seen in:

(a) Hyperthyroidism (b) Leukemia
(c) Water intoxication (d) (a) or (b) or (c)

219. Albuminocytologic dissociation in CSF is produced by:

(a) Immuno-mediated diseases (b) Neural compression
(c) Infarction (d) All of them

220. IgG index is useful for distinguishing between:

(a) Inflammatory lesions (b) Non-inflammatory lesions
(c) CSF cell counts (d) Both (a) and (b)

221. Monoclonal bands (obtained by electrophoresis of CSF protein) seen in:

(a) Multiple sclerosis (b) Neurological disease
(c) Encephalitis (d) None of them

222. In the γ-globulin region, oligoclonal bands (obtained by electrophoresis of CSF protein) are associated with:

(a) Encephalitis (b) Neurologic disease
(c) Multiple sclerosis (d) Both (a) and (c)

223. More hpatotoxicity confined to the compounds:

(a) Lipophilic (b) Hydrophilic
(c) Either (a) or (b) (d) None of them

224. Cytochrome P-450 acts on various:

(a) Carcinogens (b) Pollutants
(c) Both (a) and (b) (d) None of them

225. Acute nephrotoxicity may initially induce polyuria, followed by:

(a) Oligouria (b) Anuria
(c) Either (a) or (b) (d) Neither (a) or (b)

226. Nephrotoxic are:

(a) Hemoglobin (b) Myoglobin
(c) Bilirubin (d) Both (a) and (b)

227. The rumen of mature cattle can produce:

(a) 1.2-2.0 L gas/minute (b) 1.2- 1.8 L gas/minute
(c) 1.0- 1.5 L gas/minute (d) None of them

228. *Streptococcus bovis* is the rumen microorganism chiefly responsible for:

(a) Rapid fermentation of lactic acid

(b) Rapid production of lactic acid

(c) Both (a) and (b)

(d) None of them

229. Cardiac irregularities caused by hyperkalemia is a direct cause of death in calves with:

(a) Acute diarrhoea
(b) Marked hypoglycemia
(c) Both (a) and (b)
(d) None of them

230. In the pathogenesis of certain types of acute diarrhoea, major factor is:

(a) Increased intestinal secretion of water

(b) Increased intestinal secretion of electrolytes

(c) Both (a) and (b)

(d) None of them

231. When neutrophils attach to endothelium they release the compound, which promote extravasation:

(a) Lactoferrin
(b) Elastase
(c) Both (a) and (b)
(d) None of them

232. Depending on the duration and severity of ischemia, oxygenation of tissue is compromised and there is a subsequent attenuation of:

(a) Oxidative phosphorylation
(b) Decrease in ATP
(c) Both (a) and (b)
(d) None of them

233. Vomition results in expulsion of gastric contents caused by:

(a) Toxic irritants
(b) Infectious agents
(c) Foreign bodies
(d) All of them

234. Highest activity of gamma glutamyltransferase is found in:

(a) Renal convoluted tubular epithelium

(b) Canalicular surfaces of hepatocytes

(c) Bile duct epithelium

(d) All of them

235. The clinical signs of acute massive hepatic necrosis are:

(a) Hepatic encephalopathy

(b) Disseminated intravascular coagulopathy

(c) Edema

(d) All of them

236. Theories of toxic effects of phosphate are:

(a) Tissue calcification

(b) Increased metabolic rate by renal tubular cells

(c) Cell damage by calcium uptake

(d) All of them

237. Marked decrease in glomerular filtration rate is associated with:

(a) Oligouria (b) Anuria

(c) Either (a) or (b) (d) Neither (a) or (b)

238. The complications of oligouric or anuric renal failure:

(a) Extra renal losses (b) Fluid retention

(c) Edema (d) All of them

239. In uremia, anionic drugs have plasma protein binding:

(a) Decreased (b) Increased

(c) Normal (d) None of them

240. In uremia, cationic drugs have plasma protein binding:

(a) Normal (b) Increased

(c) Either (a) or (b) (d) Neither (a) or (b)

Answer Key

1	(c)	27	(d)	53	(a)	79	(d)
2	(b)	28	(a)	54	(d)	80	(a)
3	(c)	29	(c)	55	(a)	81	(a)
4	(c)	30	(d)	56	(c)	82	(a)
5	(a)	31	(d)	57	(a)	83	(d)
6	(c)	32	(c)	58	(a)	84	(d)
7	(b)	33	(c)	59	(a)	85	(b)
8	(a)	34	(c)	60	(d)	86	(a)
9	(a)	35	(d)	61	(d)	87	(c)
10	(b)	36	(d)	62	(d)	88	(b)
11	(c)	37	(b)	63	(b)	89	(c)
12	(d)	38	(a)	64	(c)	90	(b)
13	(a)	39	(b)	65	(a)	91	(d)
14	(d)	40	(c)	66	(c)	92	(c)
15	(c)	41	(b)	67	(c)	93	(b)
16	(b)	42	(a)	68	(b)	94	(a)
17	(d)	43	(c)	69	(a)	95	(b)
18	(b)	44	(a)	70	(b)	96	(c)
19	(a)	45	(a)	71	(a)	97	(b)
20	(a)	46	(b)	72	(d)	98	(a)
21	(a)	47	(a)	73	(a)	99	(a)
22	(a)	48	(b)	74	(a)	100	(b)
23	(c)	49	(b)	75	(a)	101	(b)
24	(b)	50	(c)	76	(d)	102	(b)
25	(d)	51	(d)	77	(c)	103	(b)
26	(b)	52	(c)	78	(d)	104	(b)

105	(a)	139	(b)	173	(d)	207	(c)
106	(b)	140	(a)	174	(d)	208	(c)
107	(b)	141	(d)	175	(d)	209	(c)
108	(a)	142	(c)	176	(c)	210	(d)
109	(c)	143	(c)	177	(c)	211	(d)
110	(a)	144	(d)	178	(d)	212	(d)
111	(d)	145	(c)	179	(a)	213	(a)
112	(c)	146	(c)	180	(d)	214	(d)
113	(a)	147	(b)	181	(c)	215	(d)
114	(a)	148	(b)	182	(d)	216	(d)
115	(a)	149	(d)	183	(c)	217	(d)
116	(a)	150	(d)	184	(c)	218	(d)
117	(a)	151	(d)	185	(c)	219	(d)
118	(c)	152	(d)	186	(d)	220	(d)
119	(c)	153	(d)	187	(d)	221	(b)
120	(a)	154	(d)	188	(d)	222	(d)
121	(a)	155	(a)	189	(d)	223	(a)
122	(a)	156	(d)	190	(c)	224	(c)
123	(a)	157	(c)	191	(c)	225	(c)
124	(d)	158	(a)	192	(c)	226	(d)
125	(a)	159	(a)	193	(c)	227	(a)
126	(b)	160	(a)	194	(d)	228	(c)
127	(c)	161	(a)	195	(d)	229	(c)
128	(c)	162	(a)	196	(d)	230	(c)
129	(a)	163	(a)	197	(d)	231	(c)
130	(a)	164	(d)	198	(c)	232	(c)
131	(a)	165	(d)	199	(d)	233	(d)
132	(d)	166	(a)	200	(d)	234	(d)
133	(d)	167	(c)	201	(a)	235	(d)
134	(a)	168	(a)	202	(d)	236	(d)
135	(d)	169	(c)	203	(d)	237	(c)
136	(a)	170	(d)	204	(c)	238	(d)
137	(c)	171	(a)	205	(c)	239	(a)
138	(a)	172	(c)	206	(d)	240	(c)

Chapter 17

Biochemistry of Diseases

1. **Genetic diseases are:**
   (a) Chromosomal disorders
   (b) Monogenic disorders
   (c) Multifactorial disorders
   (d) All of these

2. **In chromosomal disorders there is:**
   (a) Excess of chromosomes
   (b) Loss of chromosomes
   (c) Either (a) or (b)
   (d) Neither (a) or (b)

3. **Chromosomal translocations:**
   (a) Activate oncogens
   (b) Do not activate oncogens
   (c) Both (a) and (b)
   (d) None of them

4. **Monogenic disorders are:**
   (a) Autosomal dominant
   (b) Autosomal recessive
   (c) X-Linked
   (d) All of them

5. **In autosomal recessive disorder:**
   (a) One chromosome affected
   (b) Both chromosomes affected
   (c) Mutation present on x-chromosome
   (d) None of them

6. **In autosomal dominant disorder:**
   (a) Both chromosomes affected
   (b) One chromosome affected
   (c) Both (a) and (b)
   (d) None of them

7. **Females have two chromosomes, may be:**
   (a) Homozygous
   (b) Heterozygous
   (c) Either (a) or (b)
   (d) Neither (a) or (b)

8. **Under multifactorial disorders, common are:**
   (a) Ischemic heart disease
   (b) Hypertension
   (c) Both (a) and (b)
   (d) None of them

9. **In phenylketonuria, less tyrosine is synthesized, resulting in:**
   (a) Increased phenylalanine level in plasma
   (b) Increased amount of phenylpyruvate
   (c) Other metabolites of phenylalanine
   (d) All of them

10. **Phenylketonuria causes decreased availability for:**
   (a) Protein synthesis in brain
   (b) Neurotransmitter synthesis in brain
   (c) Both (a) and (b)
   (d) None of them

11. **Gene therapy could involve:**
   (a) Gene replacement
   (b) Correction
   (c) Augmentation
   (d) All of them

12. **In atherosclerosis – a slowly progressive disease, there is:**
   (a) Large to medium sized muscular arteries
   (b) Large elastic arteries
   (c) Elevated focal fibro fatty plaques
   (d) All of them

13. **In atherosclerosis, principal larger vessels affected are:**
   (a) Abdominal aorta
   (b) Descending thoracic aorta
   (c) Internal carotid arteries
   (d) All of them

14. **In atherosclerosis, medium to smaller sized vessels affected are:**
   (a) Popliteal arteries
   (b) Coronary arteries
   (c) Circles of willis in brain
   (d) All of them

15. Atherosclerosis is correlated with:

(a) Elevated LDL
(b) Inversely related to HDL level
(c) Both (a) and (b)
(d) None of them

16. Hereditary defects cause:

(a) Elevated LDL
(b) Hypercholesterolemia
(c) Accelerated atherosclerosis
(d) All of them

17. The accumulation of cholesterol in blood vessels develops, when the cholesterol synthesized by more than the amount required for the synthesis of:

(a) Membranes
(b) Bile salts
(c) Steroids
(d) All of them

18. Cholesterol synthesis is inhibited by product derived from fungi:

(a) Lovastatin
(b) Compactin
(c) Both (a) and (b)
(d) None of them

19. Lovastatin + edible resin:

(a) Prevents reabsorption from intestine
(b) Binds bile acids
(c) Both (a) and (b)
(d) None of them

20. Vitamin E has got beneficial effects in atherosclerosis due to:

(a) Inhibition of platelets aggregation
(b) Inhibition of lipid peroxide
(c) Elevation of HDL cholesterol level
(d) All of them

21. Porphyria is a metabolic disorder of heme synthesis, characterized by excretion of:

(a) Porphyrins
(b) Porphyrin precursors
(c) Either (a) or (b)
(d) Neither (a) or (b)

22. Porphyria is:

(a) Inherited
(b) Acquired
(c) Either (a) or (b)
(d) Neither (a) or (b)

23. In erythropoietic porphyria, enzyme deficiency occurs in:

(a) Liver
(b) Erythrocytes
(c) Brain
(d) None of them

24. In hepatic porphyria, enzyme deficiency occurs in:

(a) Brain
(b) Liver
(c) Erythrocytes
(d) None of them

25. Accute intermittent porphyria characterized by increased excretion of:

(a) Porphobilinogen
(b) δ-amino levulinate
(c) Both (a) and (b)
(d) None of them

26. Neuropsychiatric disturbances observed in acute intermittent porphyria results in the accumulation of:

(a) Tryptophan
(b) 5-hydroxytryptamine
(c) Both (a) and (b)
(d) None of them

27. After the administration of drugs like barbiturates, ALA synthase activity is increased, resulting in the accumulation of:

(a) PBG
(b) ALA
(c) Both (a) and (b)
(d) None of them

28. In congenital erythropoietic porphyria, there is excretion of:

(a) Uroporphyrinogen I
(b) Coproporphyrinogen I
(c) Both (a) and (b)
(d) None of them

29. Congenital erythropoietic porphyria is caused by:

(a) Autosomal recessive mode of inheritance
(b) Defect in uroporphyrinogen III cosynthase
(c) Both (a) and (b)
(d) None of them

30. In congenital erythropoietic porphyria, there is:

(a) Increased hemolysis
(b) Itching of skin
(c) Burning of skin
(d) All of them

31. Toxic porphyria is due to exposure to:

(a) Heavy metals
(b) Toxic compounds
(c) Drugs
(d) All of them

32. In toxic porphyria, there is inhibition of enzymes in heme synthesis:

(a) ALA dehydratase
(b) Uroporphyrin I synthase
(c) Ferrochelatase
(d) All of them

33. Protoporphyria caused by the:

(a) Accumulation of protoporphyrin IX (b) Deficiency of ferrochelatase

(c) Both (a) and (b) (d) None of them

34. In protoporphyria, red fluorescene is shown by:

(a) Reticulocytes (b) Skin biopsy

(c) Both (a) and (b) (d) None of them

35. Variegate porphyria is caused by:

(a) Defective protoporphyrinogen oxidase

(b) Non-production of protoporphyrin IX

(c) High concentration of coproporphyrinogen

(d) All of them

36. Hereditary coproporphyria's characters are:

(a) Defects in coproporphyrinogen oxidase

(b) Inhibition of ALA synthase

(c) Photosensitiveness

(d) All of them

37. Porphyria cutanea tarda is caused by:

(a) Deficiency of uroporphyrinogen decarboxylase

(b) Liver damage

(c) Both (a) and (b)

(d) None of them

38. Important features of porphyria cutanea tarda are:

(a) Cutaneous photosensitivity

b) Fluorescene exhibited by liver

(c) Increased excretion of uroporphyrin I and III

(d) All of them

39. In sickle cell anemia, hemoglobin has:

(a) 2 α-globin chains (normal) (b) 2 β-globin chains

(c) 2 β-globlin chains (abnormal) (d) Both (a) and (c)

40. Sickle cell anemia is due to a change in single nucleotide of:

(a) α-globin gene (b) β-globin gene

(c) Both (a) and (b) (d) None of them

41. Sickle cell anemia is heterozygous, when one gene is affected of:

(a) α-chain
(b) β-chain
(c) Both (a) and (b)
(d) None of them

42. The erythrocytes of heterozygous hemoglobin contains:

(a) HbS
(b) HbA
(c) Both (a) and (b)
(d) None of them

43. The individuals of heterozygous sickle cell anemia:

(a) Show clinical symptoms
(b) Do not show clinical symptoms
(c) Remain inert
(d) None of them

44. Sickled cells:

(a) Block the capillaries
(b) Damage to tissues
(c) Cause hemolysis
(d) All of them

45. Diabetes mellitus is caused by the deficiency in the secretion of:

(a) Glucagon
(b) Insulin
(c) Epinephrine
(d) None of them

46. Diabetes mellitus is of the type:

(a) Type I (IDDM)
(b) Type II (NIDDM)
(c) Both (a) and (b)
(d) None of them

47. IDDM requires:

(a) Insulin therapy
(b) Balance between dietary intake and insulin
(c) Both (a) and (b)
(d) None of them

48. β-cell destruction may be caused by:

(a) Drugs
(b) Viruses
(c) Autoimmunity
(d) All of them

49. Diabetic patients are unable to take up glucose efficiently from the blood, because the insulin triggers the movement of glucose transporters to the plasma membrane of:

(a) Muscle
(b) Adipose tissue
(c) Both (a) and (b)
(d) None of them

50. A characteristic metabolic change in diabetes is:

(a) Complete oxidation of fatty acid in liver

(b) Incomplete oxidation of fatty acid in liver

(c) Excessive oxidation

(d) None of them

51. The accumulation of acetyl CoA (produced by β-oxidation) leads to the over production of:

(a) Acetone bodies (b) β-hydroxybutyrate

(c) Acetoacetate (d) All of them

52. Causative factors for diabetes mellitus are:

(a) Genetic (b) Environmental

(c) Obesity (d) All of them

53. Overeating causes:

(a) Increased insulin production (b) Decreased synthesis of insulin receptors

(c) Both (a) and (b) (d) None of them

54. Biochemical indices of diabetic control are:

(a) Glycated hemoglobin (b) Serum lipids

(c) Fructosamine (d) All of them

55. Galactose metabolism is impaired leading to increased level of galactose in:

(a) Circulation (b) Urine

(c) Both (a) and (b) (d) None of them

56. The functions of liver, nervous tissue and kidneys are impaired due to the accumulation of:

(a) Galactose-1-phosphate (b) Galactitol

(c) Both (a) and (b) (d) None of them

57. Clinical symptoms of galactosemia are:

(a) Hepatospleenomegaly (b) Mental retardation

(c) Jaundice (d) All of them

58. In severe galactosemia, symptoms are:

(a) Amino aciduria (b) Albuminuria

(c) Cataract (d) All of them

59. Elevated galactose is seen in:

(a) Cirrhosis
(b) Infective hepatitis
(c) Hepato cellular damage
(d) All of them

60. Galactose is obtained by the:

(a) Hydrolysis of lactose by lactase of intestinal mucosal cells
(b) Lysosomal degradation of glycolipids and glycoproteins within the cells
(c) Both (a) and (b)
(d) None of them

61. Hypoglycemia of baby pigs is characterized by:

(a) Weakness
(b) Convulsions
(c) Coma
(d) All of them

62. The following species (new-born) can resist starvation hypoglycemia for more than a week:

(a) Lambs
(b) Calves
(c) Foals
(d) All of them

63. Starvation of new born pigs under natural conditions can occur due to the factors relating to:

(a) Agalacia
(b) Anemia
(c) Either (a) or (b)
(d) Neither (a) or (b)

64. Persistent hypoglycemia :

(a) Inhibits insulin secretion
(b) Stimulates secretion of catecholamines
(c) Both (a) and (b)
(d) None of them

65. Liver cells, intestinal mucosa and cells of renal tubular epithelium are loaded with glycogen, which is:

(a) Normal in structure
(b) Not available metabolically
(c) Both (a) and (b)
(d) None of them

66. Liver, heart and muscles are affected in:

(a) Pompe's disease
(b) Forbe's disease
(c) Anderson's disease
(d) All of them

67. Clinical features of McArdle's disease are:

(a) Muscle cramps on exercise
(b) Stiffness of muscles
(c) Weakness
(d) All of them

68. Due to impaired ability to produce glucose from glycogen, hypoglycemia is also found in some of the glycogen storage diseases:

(a) Her's disease
(b) Von Gierke's disease
(c) Both (a) and (b)
(d) None of them

69. Fasting blood glucose level may be reduced in:

(a) Addison's disease
(b) Simmond's disease
(c) Myxoedema
(d) All of them

70. The chief substrates of ruminant ketosis are:

(a) Propionate
(b) Amino acids
(c) Volatile fatty acid
(d) All of them

71. Bovine ketosis is of the types:

(a) Underfeeding ketosis
(b) Alimentary ketosis
(c) Spontaneous ketosis
(d) All of them

72. Underfeeding ketosis occurs when a dairy cow receives insufficient calories to meet:

(a) Lactational demand
(b) Body maintenance
(c) Both (a) and (b)
(d) None of them

73. Ovine pregnancy toxemia occurs in pregnant ewes subjected to:

(a) Caloric deprivation
(b) Stress
(c) Either (a) or (b)
(d) Neither (a) or (b)

74. Ovine pregnancy toxemia is characterized by depression and weakness, which is associated with:

(a) Hypoglycemia
(b) Ketonemia
(c) Ketonuria
(d) All of them

75. In ovine pregnancy toxemia, fatty acid deposition takes place in liver and impairment of liver function results in:

(a) Unable to rise
(b) Become comatose
(c) Death
(d) All of them

76. Phosphofructokinase in normal dog RBCs consists of:

(a) 86% M-type
(b) 2% L-type
(c) 12% P-type
(d) All of them

77. In dogs affected with phosphofructokinase deficiency the following results can be seen:

(a) Sub-unit composition of normal tissues

(b) Total RBC

(c) Muscle PFK activities

(d) All of them

78. Homozygously affected dogs (PFK deficiency) show:

(a) Hemolytic anemia

(b) Intravascular hemolysis with hemoglobinuria

(c) Both (a) and (b)

(d) None of them

79. Due to hemolytic crisis, dogs show:

(a) Pale mucous membrane
(b) Muscle wasting
(c) Fever as high as 41°C
(d) All of them

80. Canine skeletal muscle is less dependent on anaerobic glycolysis, so the deficient dogs show:

(a) Less evidence of myopathy
(b) More evidence of myopathy
(c) Neutral character
(d) None of them

81. Heterozygous carrier dogs have normal enzyme activity in serum approximately:

(a) One half
(b) One fourth
(c) One sixth
(d) None of them

82. The M-type sub-units at birth are:

(a) Low
(b) High
(c) Very high
(d) None of them

83. The dogs affected by pyruvate kinase deficiency die by 3 years of age due to:

(a) Bone marrow failure
(b) Liver disease
(c) Either (a) or (b)
(d) Neither (a) or (b)

84. In pyruvate kinase deficiency, homozygously affected animals show:

(a) Decreased exercise tolerance
(b) Pale mucous membrane
(c) Spleenomegaly
(d) All of them

85. Animals affected by hereditary somatocytosis have polysystemic diseases showing:

(a) Growth retardation (b) Diarrhoea
(c) Hind limb weakness (d) All of them

86. Animals affected by hereditary somatocytosis have slightly reduced:

(a) RBS counts (b) Hemoglobin values
(c) Both (a) and (b) (d) None of them

87. In hereditary somatocytosis, RBCs from all breeds have:

(a) Increased osmotic fragility (b) Shortened RBC survival
(c) Both (a) and (b) (d) None of them

88. The composition of phospholipids and cholesterol in animals affected from hereditary somatocytosis is abnormal in:

(a) Plasma (b) RBC membrane
(c) Both (a) and (b) (d) None of them

89. Iron deficiency exists in animals as:

(a) Iron deficiency (b) Iron deficient erythropoiesis
(c) Iron deficiency anemia (d) All of them

90. In iron deficiency anemia serum iron is decreased below:

(a) 50μg/dl (b) 40μg/dl
(c) 30μg/dl (d) 20μg/dl

91. Iron deficiency results from:

(a) Inadequate intake (b) Excessive loss
(c) Adequate intake (d) None of them

92. During iron deficiency:

(a) Acid secretion by stomach is reduced
(b) Intestinal absorption is impaired
(c) Both (a) and (b)
(d) None of them

93. When dietary iron is restricted, there is a fall in the activity of:

(a) Cytochrome P450 (b) Oxidative enzymes
(c) Both (a) and (b) (d) None of them

94. Iron deficiency is associated with:
- (a) Impaired cell mediated immunity
- (b) Ability of polymorphonuclear granulocytes to kill ingested bacteria
- (c) Both (a) and (b)
- (d) None of them

95. The reason for the abnormality in iron deficiency is due to:
- (a) Defective DNA synthesis
- (b) Decreased activity of ribonucleotide reductase
- (c) Both (a) and (b)
- (d) None of them

96. Altered behaviour associated with iron deficiency is:
- (a) Apathy
- (b) Irritability
- (c) Both (a) and (b)
- (d) None of them

97. Iron deficiency leads to:
- (a) Degradation of aldehyde oxidase
- (b) Elevation in the level of serotonin
- (c) Both (a) and (b)
- (d) None of them

98. α-Glycerophosphate dehydrogenase activity is reduced in iron deficiency during:
- (a) Iron depletion
- (b) Response to iron therapy
- (c) Both (a) and (b)
- (d) None of them

99. In iron deficiency, the biochemical abnormalities have been associated with physiological function for:
- (a) Central nervous system
- (b) Striated muscles
- (c) Gastrointestinal tract
- (d) All of them

100. New Hampshire chicks, when raised on iron deficient diet have:
- (a) White feathers
- (b) Reddish brown feathers
- (c) Black feathers
- (d) None of them

Answer Key

1	(d)	26	(c)	51	(d)	76	(d)		
2	(c)	27	(c)	52	(d)	77	(d)		
3	(a)	28	(c)	53	(c)	78	(c)		
4	(d)	29	(c)	54	(d)	79	(d)		
5	(b)	30	(d)	55	(c)	80	(a)		
6	(b)	31	(d)	56	(c)	81	(a)		
7	(c)	32	(d)	57	(d)	82	(a)		
8	(c)	33	(c)	58	(d)	83	(c)		
9	(d)	34	(c)	59	(d)	84	(d)		
10	(c)	35	(d)	60	(c)	85	(d)		
11	(d)	36	(d)	61	(c)	86	(c)		
12	(d)	37	(c)	62	(d)	87	(c)		
13	(d)	38	(d)	63	(c)	88	(c)		
14	(d)	39	(d)	64	(c)	89	(d)		
15	(c)	40	(b)	65	(c)	90	(a)		
16	(d)	41	(b)	66	(c)	91	(b)		
17	(d)	42	(c)	67	(c)	92	(c)		
18	(c)	43	(b)	68	(c)	93	(c)		
19	(c)	44	(d)	69	(d)	94	(c)		
20	(d)	45	(b)	70	(d)	95	(c)		
21	(c)	46	(c)	71	(d)	96	(c)		
22	(c)	47	(c)	72	(c)	97	(c)		
23	(b)	48	(d)	73	(c)	98	(c)		
24	(b)	49	(c)	74	(d)	99	(d)		
25	(c)	50	(b)	75	(d)	100	(a)		

Chapter 18

Tools of Biochemistry

1. **Chromatography is a technique by which a chemical compound is:**
   (a) Separated (b) Identified
   (c) Both (a) and (b) (d) None of them
2. **Chromatography is found useful for the:**
   (a) Fractionation of complex mixture
   (b) Separation of closely related compounds
   (c) Isolation of unstable substances (d) All of them
3. **All the chromatographic methods are similar in:**
   (a) Experimental techniques (b) Basic principles
   (c) Operating conditions (d) All of them
4. **Chromatography can be carried out by the distribution of components in a mixture between a:**
   (a) Stationary phase (b) Mobile phase
   (c) Both (a) and (b) (d) None of them
5. **In the chromatographic procedure, steps involved are:**
   (a) Preparation of stationary phase (b) Introduction of sample
   (c) Collection of components (d) All of them

6. **Solvent mobile phase should satisfy the following properties with respect tosample:**
   (a) Viscosity (b) Stability
   (c) Solubility (d) All of them

7. **Absorption is applicable for the separation of mixture of:**
   (a) Similar molecules (b) Dissimilar molecules
   (c) Both (a) and (b) (d) None of them

8. **The mobile phase consists of solvents in number:**
   (a) One (b) More than one
   (c) Both (a) and (b) (d) None of them

9. **In partition chromatography, the molecules used are:**
   (a) Non-polar (b) Less polar
   (c) Polar (d) None of them

10. **Ion-exchange chromatography helps in the separation of ions of:**
   (a) Similar properties (b) Dis-similar properties
   (c) Both (a) and (b) (d) None of them

11. **Ion-exchange chromatography is performed on the columns with:**
   (a) Adsorbent (b) Cation exchanger
   (c) Anion exchanger (d) All of them

12. **In gel chromatography, fractionation is based on the species's:**
   (a) Molecular size (b) Shape
   (c) Both (a) and (b) (d) None of them

13. **Gel chromatography is also known as:**
   (a) Gel permeation chromatography (b) Exclusion chromatography
   (c) Molecular sieve chromatography (d) All of them

14. **In gel chromatography, gel used is:**
   (a) Dexran (b) Agarose
   (c) Polyacrylamide (d) All of them

15. **Trade name for Dextran is:**
   (a) Sephadex (b) Sepharose
   (c) Bio-gel P (d) None of them

16. Agarose is a linear polymer of:

(a) D-galactose (b) 3,6-anhydro-1-Galactose

(c) Both (a) and (b) (d) None of them

17. Polyacrylamide gel is prepared by cross-linking:

(a) N, N – methylene bisacrylamide (b) Acrylamide

(c) Both (a) and (b) (d) None of them

18. In gel chromatography, separation is independent of:

(a) Temperature (b) Ionic strength

(c) pH (d) All of them

19. Gel chromatography is a valuable analytical tool in:

(a) Study of RNA metabolism

(b) Plasma protein fractionation for disease diagnosis

(c) Study of binding between protein and small molecules

(d) All of them

20. Gel chromatography is used in:

(a) Enzyme assay (b) Protein purification

(c) Synthesis of various regents (d) All of them

21. Exclusion limit of sephadex G-200 is:

(a) 8,000-10,000 (b) 3,500-4,000

(c) 2,00,000 (d) None of them

22. The more porous gel like G-75 used in the fractionation and purification of macromolecules like:

(a) Proteins (b) Nucleic acids

(c) Polysaccharides (d) All of them

23. In paper chromatography, when the movement of mobile phase is in upward direction, known as:

(a) Ascending development (b) Descending development

(c) Both (a) and (b) (d) None of them

24. In paper chromatography, the choice of paper depends on:

(a) Thickness (b) Flow rate

(c) Purity (d) All of them

25. Stationary phase used in paper chromatography are:

(a) Aqueous stationary phase (b) Hydrophilic stationary phase

(c) Hydrophobic stationary phase (d) All of them

26. Depending upon the type of complexity involved, paper chromatography may be:

(a) One dimensional (b) Two dimensional

(c) Either (a) or (b) (d) Neither (a) or (b)

27. Rate of flow (RF value) depends on:

(a) Nature of solvent (b) Temperature

(c) Nature of mixture to be separated (d) All of them

28. Adosrbent used in thin layer chromatography:

(a) Silica gel (b) Alumina

(c) Cellulose (d) All of them

29. Advantages of thin layer chromatography are:

(a) Greater resolving power

(b) Greater speed of separation

(c) Wider choice of materials as sorbents

(d) All of them

30. Thin layer chromatography constitutes a versatile analytical tool for components like:

(a) Amino acids (b) Antibiotics

(c) Dyes (d) All of them

31. Affinity chromatography is useful for the separation of:

(a) Enzymes (b) Glycoproteins

(c) Nucleic acids (d) All of them

32. High pressure liquid chromatography (HPLC) is more advantageous for the separation of:

(a) Large molecules (b) Non-volatile compounds

(c) Thermolabile compounds (d) All of them

33. Advantages of high pressure liquid chromatography:

(a) High resolving power

(b) Accurate quantitative measurement

(c) Repetitive and reproducible analysis

(d) All of them

34. HPLC can be applied for the:

(a) Separation of lipids
(b) Separation of steroids
(c) Separation of coal and oil products
(d) All of them

35. In adsorption chromatography stationary phase is:

(a) Solid
(b) Liquid
(c) Gas
(d) All of them

36. Solubility is greatly affected by:

(a) H-bonds
(b) Dipole interaction
(c) Charge transfer
(d) All of them

37. Thin layer chromatography requires less substance than:

(a) Paper chromatography
(b) Column chromatography
(c) Both (a) and (b)
(d) None of them

38. The columns in ion-exchange chromatography may be operated in:

(a) Elution
(b) Frontal analysis
(c) Displacement
(b) All of them

39. In gas chromatography distribution of gaseous solutes takes place between a:

(a) Gas and a liquid
(b) Gas and a solid
(c) Either (a) or (b)
(d) Neither (a) or (b)

40. The term chromatography was first developed by:

(a) Mikhail Tswett
(b) Kirland and Huber
(c) Karl Runge
(d) None of them

41. In HPLC maximum temperature is:

(a) 80°C
(b) 120°C
(c) 100°C
(d) 140°C

42. pH meter is an electrochemical device and makes use of:

(a) Glass electrode
(b) Calomel electrode
(c) Both (a) and (b)
(d) None of them

43. Physical absorption when compared with chemisorption is:

(a) Weaker (b) Stronger
(c) Equivalent (d) None of them

44. Electrode sensitive to hydrogen ions is:

(a) Glass electrode (b) Calomel electrode
(c) Either (a) or (b) (d) Neither (a) or (b)

45. Electrophoresis is applied to the migration of:

(a) Individual ions (b) Colloidal aggregates
(c) Both (a) and (b) (d) None of them

46. The movement of charged substances depends on:

(a) Ionic strength of solution (b) Charge of substance
(c) Size of molecule (d) All of them

47. The electrophoretic separation of the sample is affected by:

(a) pH (b) Buffer
(c) Voltage (d) All of them

48. In electrophoresis, when the separation is carried out in presence of supporting medium, known as:

(a) Zone electrophoresis (b) Ionophoresis
(c) Electromigration (d) All of them

49. In zone electrophoresis, separation depends on the properties of media. The media used are:

(a) Cellulose acetate strips (b) Starch powder
(c) Agarose gel (d) All of them

50. Paper electrophoresis can be applied for the fractionation of:

(a) Alkaloids (b) Antibiotics
(c) Vitamins (d) All of them

51. Paper electrophoresis is used in the analysis of:

(a) Serum (b) Urine
(c) Gastric juice (d) All of them

52. Electrophoresis on cellulose acetate gives better resolution than paper electrophoresis, because cellulose acetate:

(a) Stabilizes fluids more efficiently (b) More homogenous
(c) Both (a) and (b) (d) None of them

53. Isotachophoresis has been used to separate complex mixtures of:

(a) Proteins
(b) Small ions
(c) Fatty acids
(d) All of them

54. In polyacrylamide gel, denaturant used is:

(a) Urea
(b) Calcium sulphate
(c) Potassium sulphate
(d) None of them

55. The advantages of polyacrylamide gel electrophoresis are:

(a) Better resolution
(b) can be used with wide variety of buffer
(c) Causes no electro-endosmotic effect
(d) All of them

56. In agarose gel electrophoresis, larger molecules migrate:

(a) Slowly
(b) At a faster rate
(c) Very fast
(d) None of them

57. There is a linear relationship between the:

(a) Log of electrophoretic mobility of DNA
(b) Gel concentration
(c) Both (a) and (b)
(d) None of them

58. Through the agar gel, the migration is at different rates for the DNAs form:

(a) Superhelical circular (Form I)
(b) Nicked circular (Form II)
(c) Linear (Form III)
(d) All of them

59. The relative mobilities of the three forms of DNA depend on the:

(a) Concentration
(b) Type of agarose for gel
(c) Both (a) and (b)
(d) None of them

60. The relative mobilities of three forms of DNA are influenced by the:

(a) Strength of applied current
(b) Ionic strength of buffer
(c) Both (a) and (b)
(d) None of them

61. Addition of ethidium bromide to gel in agarose gel electrophoresis causes:

(a) Decrease in negative charge of DNA
(b) Increase in stiffness of DNA
(c) Increase in length of DNA
(d) All of them

62. The range of separation in agarose gel decreases as the:
(a) Voltage increased
(b) Voltage decreased
(c) Remains stationary
(d) None of them

63. In agarose gel electrophoresis, gel loading buffer is used to:
(a) Increase the density of sample
(b) To add colour to get sample
(c) Both (a) and (b)
(d) None of them

64. The monomers acrylamide and bis-acrylamide are highly poisonous, but after polymerization, the product is:
(a) Toxic
(b) Non-toxic
(c) Extremely toxic
(d) None of them

65. The paper used in paper electrophoresis is:
(a) Whatman filter paper No. 1
(b) Whatman filter paper No. 2
(c) Whatman filter paper No. 3
(d) All of them

66. In electrophoresis, better separations can be achieved by using buffer, which is:
(a) Strongly acidic
(b) Strongly alkaline
(c) Either (a) or (b)
(d) Neither (a) or (b)

67. When the separation is carried out in presence of supporting medium such as paper, the technique is known as:
(a) Zone electrophoresis
(b) Electro chromatography
(c) Either (a) or (b)
(d) Neither (a) or (b)

68. Weakly acidic organic substances such as carboxylic acids and phenols are best separated at:
(a) Low pH
(b) High pH
(c) Very low pH
(d) Very high pH

69. In gas chromatography, number of theoritical plates increase with a:
(a) Decrease in particle size
(b) Increase in surface area
(c) Either (a) or (b)
(d) Neither (a) or (b)

70. The solvent used for extraction must have low:
(a) Inflammability
(b) Viscosity
(c) Both (a) and (b)
(d) None of them

71. Flame photometry or emission spectroscopy is an instrumental approach for the determination of:

(a) Alkali (b) Alkaline earth metals

(c) Both (a) and (b) (d) None of them

72. The basic instrument used for observing emission from flame consists of:

(a) Flame (b) Monochromator

(c) Detector (d) None of them

73. In flame photometry, there are some interferences:

(a) Chemical (b) Spectral

(c) Both (a) and (b) (d) None of them

74. Flame photometry depends on the number of atoms in:

(a) Ground state (b) Excited state

(c) Both (a) and (b) (d) None of them

75. Emission flame photometry depends on the number of atoms in:

(a) Excited state (b) Ground state

(c) Either (a) or (b) (d) Neither (a) or (b)

76. Source of flame in flame photometry is:

(a) Gas flow regulator (b) An atomizer

(c) Burner (d) All of them

77. The flame in flame photometry to be used for a particular analysis depends on:

(a) Temperature at which elements best excited

(b) Degree to which constituents of sample interfere with excitation

(c) Reacting species in the flame

(d) All of them

78. In flame photometry, air acetylene flame is more suitable for:

(a) Calcium (b) Magnesium

(c) Alkaline earth metals (d) All of them

79. In flame photometry air-coal gas used for:

(a) Calcium (b) Alkali metals

(c) Both (a) and (b) (d) None of them

80. In flame photometry, rich flame is used for:

(a) Barium (b) Calcium

(c) Magnesium (d) All of them

81. The temperature in air-acetylene flame is:

(a) 2200-3000°C (b) 1800-1900°C

(c) 1700-1800°C (d) None of them

82. The better sensitivity of flame can be obtained by the use of organic solvents, which:

(a) Increase the sensitivity of flame (b) Increase chance of interference

(c) Both (a) and (b) (d) None of them

83. The detectors used in flame photometry are:

(a) Photomultiplier tubes (b) Vaccum phototubes

(c) Either (a) or (b) (d) Neither (a) or (b)

84. Flame photometers are liable to show 'drift', which may be:

(a) A change in zero (b) A change in sensitivity

(c) Either (a) or (b) (d) Neither (a) or (b)

85. Zero drift in flame photometry may arise from:

(a) Change in temperature of electronic components

(b) Change in external light near the instrument

(c) Accumulation of light emitting material on burner

(d) All of them

86. Flame photometry widely used for the determination of Na and K in:

(a) Water (b) Cement

(c) Glass (d) All of them

87. Fluorescent intensity measurement permits the quantitative determination of traces of:

(a) Inorganic species (b) Organic species

(c) Both (a) and (b) (d) None of them

88. A colorimetric procedure ionvolves the following operations:

(a) Preparation of coloured solution (b) Obtaining a suitable standard

(c) Colour matching (d) All of them

89. In colorimeter, choice of an appropriate filter depends upon the:

(a) Wave length of exciting mercury lines

(b) Wave length of emitted light

(c) Both (a) and (b)

(d) None of them

90. Fluorometers may be:

(a) Single beam type
(b) Double beam type
(c) Both (a) or (b)
(d) None of them

91. Fluorometer characteristics affect:

(a) Sensitivity
(b) Precision
(c) Both (a) and (b)
(d) None of them

92. Fluorometry is more specific than spectrophotometry due to the choice of wavelength for:

(a) Radiation emitted
(b) Light exciting it
(c) Both (a) and (b)
(d) None of them

93. The ultra violet light in fluorometry used for excitation may cause:

(a) Destruction of fluorescent molecules
(b) Photochemical changes
(c) Either (a) and (b)
(d) Neither (a) or (b)

94. The presence of dissolved oxygen in fluorometry may cause:

(a) Increased photochemical destruction

(b) Reduction of fluorescent intensity

(c) Either (a) or (b)

(b) Neither (a) or (b)

95. The shift in absorption maxima occurs due to the interaction of haemoglobin with:

(a) O_2
(b) CO
(c) Some drugs
(d) All of them

96. Range of visible region is:

(a) 3800-7600 Å
(b) Below 3800 Å
(c) Above 7600 Å
(d) None of them

97. The frequency of electromagnetic radiation is:

(a) Number of waves/second
(b) Distance travelled/second
(c) Both (a) and (b)
(d) None of them

98. If a substance shows a colour in white light, colour indicates the light, which was:

(a) Absorbed
(b) Not absorbed
(c) Both (a) and (b)
(d) None of them

99. In visible region, substances used can be:

(a) Coloured
(b) Colourless
(c) Both (a) and (b)
(d) None of them

100. Approximate wave length (mμ) range for blue colour is:

(a) 465-482
(b) 487-493
(c) 571-576
(d) 597-617

101. The proportion of incident light transmitted by a solution containing light absorbing material depends on:

(a) Nature of substance
(b) Wavelength of light
(c) Amount of light absorbing material in the light path
(d) All of them

102. When a ray of monochromatic light passes through on absorbing medium, intensity decreases with an increase in:

(a) Concentration of absorbing medium
(b) Length of absorbing medium
(c) Both (a) and (b)
(d) None of them

103. In colorimetric analysis, the transmitted colour intensity is directly proportional to:

(a) Concentration of light absorbing substance
(b) Depth of solution through which light passes
(c) Both (a) and (b)
(d) None of them

104. Beer's law is not valid when:

(a) Absorbing material is coagulated
(b) Presence of impurities
(c) Suspension is there
(d) All of them

105. The instrument used for measuring coloured solution consists of:

(a) Source of radiant energy
(b) Monochromator
(c) Photometer
(d) All of them

106. Source of radiant energy is incandescent tungsten filament, the emitting capacity of which depends on:

(a) Temperature of the filament

(b) Wave length of radiant energy emitted

(c) Both (a) and (b)

(d) None of them

107. Increasing the operating temperature of filament:

(a) Wavelength maximum lowered (b) Energy output increased

(c) Lamp life shortened (d) All of them

108. In spectrophotometry, for ultraviolet work, lamp used is:

(a) High pressure hydrogen (b) Deuterium discharge lamp

(c) Either (a) or (b) (d) Neither (a) or (b)

109. In spectrophotometer, a monochromator consists of:

(a) Entrance slit (b) Exit slit

(c) A dispersing device (d) All of them

110. For the accurate determination of absorbance, mandatory are:

(a) Narrow band width (b) Continuous wave length selection

(c) Both (a) and (b) (d) None of them

111. Properties of a coloured system suitable for measurement of:

(a) Sensitivity (b) Specificity

(c) Stability (d) All of them

112. Due to the presence of heme group in hemoproteins, they absorb in:

(a) UV region (b) Visible region

(c) Both (a) and (b) (d) None of them

113. The most important dispersing devices are:

(a) Prism (b) Gratings

(c) Both (a) and (b) (d) None of them

114. Fluorescence is not shown by:

(a) Pyridine (b) Furan

(c) Pyrrole (d) All of them

115. Ultracentrifugation is an indispensable tool for the isolation of:

(a) Subcellular organelles (b) Proteins

(c) Nucleic acids (d) All of them

116. The rate at which sedimentation occurs in ultracentrifugation depends on the:

(a) Size of particles (b) Shape of particles

(c) Both (a) and (b) (d) None of them

117. In ultracentrifugation, the cells are subjected to disruption by:

(a) Sonication (b) Osmotic shock

(c) Homogenization (d) Either (a) or (b) or (c)

118. In ultracentrifugation, the fractions separated are:

(a) Nuclear (b) Mitochondrial

(c) Microsomal (d) All of them

119. The mitochondrial fraction includes:

(a) Lysosomes (b) Peroxisomes

(c) Both (a) and (b) (d) None of them

120. Purity of sub cellular fractionation is checked by the use of marker enzymes like:

(a) DNA polymerase (b) Glucose-6-phosphatase

(c) Glutamate dehydrogenase (d) All of them

121. The microsomal fraction includes:

(a) Ribosomes (b) Endoplasmic reticulum

(c) Both (a) and (b) (d) None of them

122. With a reduction in the mass of mechanical components of balance, sensitivity:

(a) Increases (b) Decreases

(c) Remains same (d) None of them

123. In case of glass electrode in pH meter, the following do not affect the potential:

(a) Salt (b) Proteins

(c) Both (a) and (b) (d) None of them

124. An analytical balance is judged on the basis of:

(a) Displacement

(b) Deflection of beam produced by unit weight

(c) Either (a) or (b)

(d) Neither (a) or (b)

125. Glass electrode in pH meter is disadvantageous, because it is:

(a) Mechanically fragile

(b) High internal resistance of glass membrane

(c) Both (a) and (b)

(d) None of them

Answer Key

1	(c)	26	(c)	51	(d)	76	(d)
2	(d)	27	(d)	52	(c)	77	(d)
3	(d)	28	(d)	53	(d)	78	(d)
4	(c)	29	(d)	54	(a)	79	(c)
5	(d)	30	(d)	55	(d)	80	(d)
6	(d)	31	(d)	56	(a)	81	(a)
7	(a)	32	(d)	57	(c)	82	(c)
8	(b)	33	(d)	58	(d)	83	(c)
9	(c)	34	(d)	59	(c)	84	(c)
10	(a)	35	(a)	60	(c)	85	(d)
11	(d)	36	(d)	61	(d)	86	(d)
12	(c)	37	(c)	62	(a)	87	(c)
13	(d)	38	(d)	63	(c)	88	(d)
14	(d)	39	(c)	64	(b)	89	(c)
15	(a)	40	(a)	65	(d)	90	(c)
16	(c)	41	(b)	66	(c)	91	(c)
17	(c)	42	(c)	67	(c)	92	(c)
18	(d)	43	(a)	68	(b)	93	(c)
19	(d)	44	(a)	69	(c)	94	(c)
20	(d)	45	(c)	70	(c)	95	(d)
21	(c)	46	(d)	71	(c)	96	(a)
22	(d)	47	(d)	72	(d)	97	(a)
23	(a)	48	(d)	73	(c)	98	(b)
24	(d)	49	(d)	74	(a)	99	(a)
25	(d)	50	(d)	75	(a)	100	(a)

101	**(d)**	**108**	**(d)**	**115**	**(d)**	**122**	**(a)**
102	**(c)**	**109**	**(d)**	**116**	**(c)**	**123**	**(c)**
103	**(c)**	**110**	**(c)**	**117**	**(d)**	**124**	**(c)**
104	**(d)**	**111**	**(d)**	**118**	**(d)**	**125**	**(c)**
105	**(d)**	**112**	**(c)**	**119**	**(b)**		
106	**(c)**	**113**	**(c)**	**120**	**(d)**		
107	**(d)**	**114**	**(d)**	**121**	**(c)**		

Chapter 19

Advanced Techniques for Biochemical Investigation

1. **Radio-immuno assay is highly:**
   (a) Sensitive (b) Specific
   (c) Both (a) and (b) (d) None of them
2. **The principle of radio-immuno assay (RIA) is based on the competition between:**
   (a) Labelled antigen (b) Unlabelled antigen
   (c) Both (a) and (b) (d) None of them
3. **As the concentration of unlabelled antigen increases, the amount of labelled antigen-antibody complex:**
   (a) Decreases (b) Increases
   (c) Remains stationary (d) None of them
4. **Radio-immuno assay has tremendous applications in the diagnosis of:**
   (a) Hormonal disorders (b) Cancer
   (c) Therapeutic monitoring of drugs (d) None of them
5. **When the substance to be analyzed is in very low concentration, method most suitable is:**
   (a) Colorimetric (b) Gravimetric
   (c) Radio-immuno assay (d) None of them

6. **Automation to the routine biochemical analysis of samples of blood or serum can be analyzed by the use of:**
   (a) Autoanalyser (b) Dialyser
   (c) Potentiometer (d) None of them

7. **Mass spectrometry provides a wealth of information for:**
   (a) Proteomics research (b) Enzymology
   (c) Protein chemistry (d) All of them

8. **Once the mass of a particular protein is known, mass spectrometry is convenient and accurate method for detecting changes in mass due to the presence of:**
   (a) Bound factors (b) Bound metal ions
   (c) Covalent modifications (d) All of them

9. **Nuclear magnetic resonance (NMR) is carried out on**
   (a) Macromolecules in solution (b) Crystallizable molecules
   (c) Both (a) and (b) (d) None of them

10. **X-ray crystallography is carried out on:**
    (a) Molecules which can be crystallized (b) Macromolecules in solution
    (c) Either (a) or (b) (d) Neither (a) or (b)

11. **Nuclear magnetic resonance can also illuminate the dynamic side of protein including:**
    (a) Conformational changes (b) Protein folding
    (c) Interaction with other molecules (d) All of them

12. **Nuclear magnetic resonance signal is given by certain atoms:**
    (a) ^{1}H (b) ^{13}C
    (c) ^{15}N (d) All of them

13. **The rapid increase in the availability of structural information about the macromolecules of living cells is possible by:**
    (a) X-ray crystallography (b) Nuclear magnetic resonance
    (c) Both (a) and (b) (d) None of them

14. **^{1}H is particularly important in NMR experiments due to its:**
    (a) High sensitivity (b) Natural abundance
    (c) Both (a) and (b) (d) None of them

15. When a strong, static magnetic field is applied to a solution containing single type of macromolecule, magnetic dipoles are aligned in the field in the orientation:

(a) Parallel
(b) Antiparallel
(c) Either (a) or (b)
(d) Neither (a) or (b)

16. By X-ray diffraction, following can be analyzed:

(a) Spacing of different kinds of atoms in complex organic molecules
(b) Proteins
(c) Both (a) and (b)
(d) None of them

17. The spacing of atoms in a crystal lattice can be determined by measuring the:

(a) Location of spots
(b) Intensities of spot
(c) Both (a) and (b)
(d) None of them

18. Radio-immuno assay is useful in diagnosing:

(a) Sex hormone sensitive tumors
(b) Insulinomas
(c) Both (a) and (b)
(d) None of them

19. Radio-immuno assay is employed for the estimation of hormones like:

(a) Insulin
(b) Thyroxine
(c) Cortisol
(d) All of them

20. Radio-immuno assay is helpful in estimating drugs like:

(a) Digoxin
(b) Digitoxin
(c) Both (a) and (b)
(d) None of them

21. Enzyme immuno assay (EIA) is classified into:

(a) Homogenous enzyme immuno assay
(b) Heterogenous enzyme immuno assay or enzyme linked immuno sorbent assay (ELISA)
(c) Both (a) and (b)
(d) None of them

22. Homogenous enzyme immuno assay is applicable for:

(a) T_3
(b) T_4
(c) Estriol
(d) All of them

23. Homogenous enzyme immuno assay couples the:

(a) Immunology (b) Enzymology

(c) Photometry (d) All of them

24. In heterogenous enzyme immuno assay, a competition is held for the antibody sites between:

(a) Unlabelled antigen (b) Labelled antigen

(c) Both (a) and (b) (d) None of them

25. The most commonly used pregnancy test for the detection of human chorionic gonadotropin (HCG) in urine is based on:

(a) ELISA (b) RIA

(c) Ultracentrifugation (d) None of them

26. Advantages of mass spectroscopy are:

(a) High precision

(b) Measurement of molecular weight

(c) Determination of constitution of pure and mixed samples

(d) All of them

27. Mass spectroscopy is more important than:

(a) Infrared

(b) Nuclear magnetic resonance spectroscopy

(c) Either (a) or (b)

(d) Neither (a) or (b)

28. Mass spectrometer is an instrument, which produces charged ions consisting of:

(a) Parent ions

(b) Ionic fragments of original molecule

(c) Both (a) and (b)

(d) None of them

29. Mass spectrometer performs following functions:

(a) Ionisation of sample

(b) Acceleration of the ions by electric field

(c) Dispersion of ions according to their mass/charge ratio

(d) All of them

30. The mass spectrum is obtained, when vapor pressure is:

(a) Higher (b) Lower

(c) Remains stationary (d) None of them

31. In mass spectrometry generally ionized ions are:

(a) Positive (b) Negative

(c) Both (a) and (b) (d) None of them

32. All organic compounds having an even molecular weight must contain number of nitrogen:

(a) Zero (b) Even

(c) Either (a) or (b) (d) Neither (a) or (b)

33. In mass spectroscopy, principle of double focusing means:

(a) Direction (b Velocity

(c) Both (a) and (b) (d) None of them

34. When a molecule or ion contains odd number of nitrogen atoms, it will have the molecular weight of value:

(a) Odd (b) Even

(c) Either (a) or (b) (d) Neither (a) or (b)

35. The molecular ion is formed by the removal of electron from the molecule of:

(a) Highest ionization potential (b) Lowest ionization potential

(c) Both (a) and (b) (d) None of them

36. Higher the electronegativity of the atom, de-shielding caused to proton is :

(a) Greater (b) Lesser

(c) No effect (d) None of them

37. The high resolution ^{14}N-NMR spectra of NH_4^+ consists of a:

(a) Quintet (b) Doublet

(c) Triplet (d) None of them

38. ^{14}N contains atomic number:

(a) Odd (b) Even

(c) Both (a) and (b) (b) None of them

39. ^{13}C contains mass number:

(a) Even (b) Odd

(c) Either (a) or (b) (d) Neither (a) or (b)

40. Radioactivity is the process of decay of unstable atomic nuclei and usually produces:

(a) Ionising radiation (b) Large amount of energy

(c) Both (a) and (b) (d) None of them

41. Radioactivity is independent of:

(a) Temperature (b) Light

(c) Magnetism (d) All of them

42. The radioactive elements range from atomic number:

(a) 83 to 92 (b) 83 to 95

(c) 83 to 98 (d) None of them

43. Atom consists of atomic particles grouped into:

(a) Negatively charged electrons (b) Positively charged protons

(c) Neutrons (d) All of them

44. Isotopes of an element are the atoms that have the nuclei with:

(a) Same number of protons (b) Same number of neutrons

(c) Same atomic number (d) None of them

45. An isotope is symbolized by the symbol of its element with mass number in:

(a) Sub-script (b) Super-script

(c) Both (a) and (b) (d) None of them

46. Radio-isotopes are:

(a) Unstable (b) Stable

(c) Partially stable (d) None of them

47. Half-life of radioactive element is the time during which the value of radioactivity falls from initial value to:

(a) Zero (b) Half of that

(c) ¼ of that (d) None of them

48. Radioactivity can be detected and measured by:

(a) Autoradiography (b) Geiger Muller

(c) Liquid scintillation counter (d) All of them

49. ^{135}I is used for thyroid function test in:

(a) Hypothyroidism (b) Hyperthyroidism

(c) Both (a) and (b) (d) None of them

50. Radio-labelled nucleotides are used in the study of:

(a) DNA or RNA sequencing (b) Replication

(c) Transcription (d) All of them

51. Auto-antibodies are the antibodies that react with antigens of:

(a) Same individual (b) Different individual

(c) Either (a) or (b) (d) Neither (a) or (b)

52. Auto-antibodies produce auto-immune disorders like:

(a) Diabetes mellitus (b) Rheumatoid arthritis

(c) Primary biliary cirrhosis (d) All of them

53. Lymphocytes are the cells which are associated with:

(a) Development of specific immune response

(b) Maintenance of specific immune response

(c) Both (a) and (b)

(d) None of them

54. Immuno assays are employed for:

(a) Diagnosis and prognosis

(b) To know the contamination of environment by pesticides

(c) Contamination of environment by toxic factors

(d) All of them

55. Radio immuno assay offers an estimation of concentrations to the level of:

(a) Micrograms (b) Pico-grams

(c) Both (a) and (b) (d) None of them

56. Enzyme linked immunosorbent assay (ELISA) does not require radioactive substances for labelling, so they are:

(a) Dangerous

(b) Restricted to authorized laboratories

(c) Either (a) or (b)

(d) Neither (a) or (b)

57. In comparison to RIA, ELISA is:

(a) Simpler
(b) Less time consuming
(c) Both (a) and (b)
(d) None of them

58. ELISA techniques widely applied for assay of:

(a) Bacterial or viral antigens
(b) Tumor marker
(c) Growth factors
(d) All of them

59. Immunophenotyping technique serves to:

(a) Identify specific kinds of cells
(b) Enumerate specific kinds of cells
(c) Both (a) and (b)
(d) None of them

60. Washing solution in ELISA is:

(a) PBS
(b) Tris buffer
(c) PBS-Tween
(d) PBS-conjugate

61. Coating buffer pH of ELISA is:

(a) 7.0
(b) 8.0
(c) 9.0
(d) 9.6

62. ABTS is the substrate of _____ enzyme in ELISA:

(a) Peroxidase
(b) β-galactosidase
(c) Alkaline phosphatase
(d) None of them

63. In indirect ELISA brucella specific antibodies are detected in sheep with _____ peroxidase conjugate:

(a) Antibovine IgG
(b) Antigoat IgG
(c) Anti sheep IgG
(d)None of them

64. Dot immunobinding assay is based on the principles of:

(a) RIA
(b) ELISA
(c) Nucleic acid hybridization
(d) None of them

65. Sandwich ELISA is performed for detection of:

(a) Antigen
(b) Antibody
(c) Both (a) and (b)
(d) None of them

66. Substrate used in DIA is:

(a) DAB
(b) OPD
(c) ABTS
(d) 5-aminosalicylic acid

67. Dot immunobinding assay can be employed in the detection of:

(a) Antibodies (b) Antigen

(c) Both (a) and (b) (d) None of them

68. Dot-ELISA can be employed for _____ detection of aflatoxin in feed:

(a) Qualitative (b) Quantitative

(c) Both (a) and (b) (d) None of them

69. ELISA is used for:

(a) Diagnosis of infectious disease

(b) Confirmation of infectious disease

(c) Both (a) and (b)

(d) None of them

70. In radio immuno assay the use of radio isotope labelled antibodies or antigen are:

(a) Hazardous to health

(b) Requires costly Y or B counter

(c) Both (a) and (b)

(d) None of them

71. ELISA is used for the detection of:

(a) Antigens (b) Antibodies

(c) Both (a) and (b) (d) None of them

72. The time required for ELISA is less due to:

(a) Use of automated dispensing (b) Washing

(c) Photometric methods (d) All of them

73. ELISA can also be used for the diagnosis of:

(a) Bacterial diseases (b) Viral diseases

(c) Parasitic diseases (d) All of them

74. The popularity of ELISA is primarily due to its:

(a) High sensitivity (b) Excellent specificity

(c) Simplicity (d) All of them

75. Many infectious diseases are diagnosed by:

(a) Isolating (b) Growing

(c) Identifying the infectious agent (d) All of them

76. Reagents for ELISA are relatively:

(a) Cheap (b) Stable

(c) Easy to prepare (d) All of them

77. Dot immunobinding assay is as good as ELISA for diagnosing:

(a) Infectious diseases (b) Non-infectious diseases

(c) Both (a) and (b) (d) None of them

78. Dot immunobinding assay could be developed to detect:

(a) Antibody in serum sample (b) Antigen in clinical sample

(c) Either (a) or (b) (d) Neither (a) or (b)

79. As the sensitivity of an assay increases, the specificity of assay:

(a) Increases (b) Decreases

(c) Remains same (d) None of them

80. Dot immunobinding assay diagnoses infectious diseases by:

(a) Detecting the presence of antibodies

(b) Detecting the presence of etiological agent

(c) Either (a) or (b)

(d) Neither (a) or (b)

81. Dye used in immunofluorescence test is:

(a) FITC (b) Rhodamine

(c) Both (a) and (b) (d) None of them

82. Slides prepared in immunofluorescence test can be stored for:

(a) One week (b) One month

(c) One day (d) One year

83. Substrate used in immuno peroxidase test for detection of antigen on tissue section is:

(a) OPD (b) DAB

(c) ABTS (d) None of them

84. Fluorescent probes:

(a) Detect rapid biochemical changes (b) Give instanteous report

(c) Both (a) and (b) (d) None of them

85. Fluorescent probes are derived from green fluorescent protein, which is:

(a) 11 stranded B-barrel

(b) Light absorbing centre of proton

(c) Light emitting centre of proton

(d) All of them

86. Fluorescent hybrid proteins used to measure:

(a) Distance between interacting components within a cell

(b) Total concentrations of compounds

(c) Both (a) and (b)

(d) None of them

87. Whenever, in the cell cAMP increases, R_2C_2 complex dissociates into:

(a) R_2 and 2C

(b) FRET signal test

(c) Both (a) and (b)

(d) None of them

88. The efficiency of Flourescence Resonance Energy Transfer (FRET) is _____ to 6th power of distance between donor and acceptor:

(a) Directly proportional

(b) Inversely proportional

(c) Either (a) or (b)

(d) Neither (a) or (b)

89. An excited fluorescent molecule can dispose energy from absorbed photon by:

(a) Fluorescence

(b) Non-radiative fluorescence energy transfer

(c) Both (a) and (b)

(d) None of them

90. Mass spectrometry can also be used to:

(a) Sequence short stretches of polypeptide

(b) Quickly identify unknown proteins

(c) Both (a) and (b)

(d) None of them

91. Clinical applications of flow cytometry are:

(a) HIV infection

(b) Stem cell enumeration

(c) Acute leukemia

(d) All of them

92. Immunophenotyping can distinguish between:

(a) Lymphoblastic (ALL) (b) Myeloblastic (AML) forms
(c) Both (a) and (b) (d) None of them

93. Analysis of _____ harvests for the number of CD 34+ cells is a useful tool for stem cell content:

(a) Bone marrow (b) Peripheral stem cells
(c) Either (a) or (b) (d) Neither (a) or (b)

94. By the help of flow cytometry many clinical disorders can be:

(a) Diagnosed (b) Managed
(c) Both (a) and (b) (b) None of them

95. By immunophenotyping, specific kinds of cells can be:

(a) Identified (b) Innumerated
(c) Both (a) and (b) (d) None of them

96. RIA techniques have been developed for:

(a) Hormones (b) Steroid
(c) Peptide in serum (d) All of them

97. In competitive binding immunoassay the amount of labeled antigen present in antibody bound antigen is determined by:

(a) Liquid scintillation for β-emission (b) γ-counter
(c) Either (a) or (b) (d) Neither (a) or (b)

98. The bound antigen is _____ to free antigen concentration in a given sample:

(a) Directly proportional (b) Inversely proportional
(c) Similar (d) None of them

99. Radio-immuno assay technique was developed by:

(a) Rosalyn Yalow (b) Samuel Berson
(c) Both (a) and (b) (d) None of them

100. Radio-immunoassay employed for variety of other purposes:

(a) Contamination of environment by pesticides
(b) Other toxic effluents from various industries
(c) Both (a) and (b)
(d) None of them

Answer Key

1	(c)	26	(d)	51	(a)	76	(d)
2	(c)	27	(c)	52	(d)	77	(c)
3	(a)	28	(c)	53	(c)	78	(c)
4	(d)	29	(d)	54	(d)	79	(b)
5	(c)	30	(a)	55	(c)	80	(c)
6	(a)	31	(a)	56	(d)	81	(c)
7	(d)	32	(c)	57	(c)	82	(a)
8	(d)	33	(c)	58	(d)	83	(b)
9	(a)	34	(a)	59	(c)	84	(c)
10	(a)	35	(b)	60	(c)	85	(d)
11	(d)	36	(a)	61	(d)	86	(c)
12	(d)	37	(a)	62	(a)	87	(c)
13	(c)	38	(a)	63	(c)	88	(b)
14	(c)	39	(c)	64	(d)	89	(c)
15	(c)	40	(c)	65	(a)	90	(c)
16	(c)	41	(d)	66	(a)	91	(d)
17	(c)	42	(a)	67	(c)	92	(c)
18	(c)	43	(d)	68	(c)	93	(c)
19	(d)	44	(a)	69	(c)	94	(c)
20	(c)	45	(b)	70	(c)	95	(c)
21	(c)	46	(a)	71	(c)	96	(d)
22	(d)	47	(b)	72	(d)	97	(c)
23	(d)	48	(d)	73	(d)	98	(b)
24	(c)	49	(c)	74	(d)	99	(c)
25	(a)	50	(d)	75	(d)	100	(c)

Chapter 20

Diagnostic Biochemistry

1. **Impairment of organ function and influence on the health is due to abnormality in the tissues caused by:**
   (a) Exogenous factors (b) Endogenous factors
   (c) Both (a) and (b) (d) None of them

2. **Liver participates in the metabolism of:**
   (a) Carbohydrate (b) Lipid
   (c) Protein (d) All of them

3. **Liver participates in the:**
   (a) Formation of blood (b) Synthesis of plasma proteins
   (c) Destruction of erythrocytes (d) All of them

4. **Liver can store:**
   (a) Glycogen (b) Vitamin A
   (c) Iron (d) All of them

5. **Liver function tests helps in the:**
   (a) Detection of abnormality
   (b) Detection of extent of liver damage
   (c) Capacity of liver to perform the functions
   (d) All of them

6. The tests based on synthetic functions are:

(a) Prothrombin time (b) Serum albumin
(c) Both (a) and (b) (d) None of them

7. Tests based on excretory functions are:

(a) Measurement of bile pigments (b) Measurement of bile salts
(c) Measurement of Bromosulphthalein (d) All of them

8. Tests based on serum enzymes derived from liver:

(a) Determination of transaminases
(b) Determination of alkaline phosphatase
(c) Determination of 5–nucleotidase
(d) All of them

9. Tests based on metabolic capacity are:

(a) Galactose tolerance (b) Antipyrine clearance
(c) Both (a) and (b) (d) None of them

10. Vanden Bergh reaction given by normal serum is:

(a) Positive (b) Negative
(c) Either (a) or (b) (d) Neither (a) or (b)

11. Type of jaundice is characterized by increased serum concentration of:

(a) Unconjugated bilirubin (b) Conjugated bilirubin
(c) Both (a) and (b) (d) None of them

12. Conjugated bilirubin:

(a) Excreted in urine (b) Not excreted in urine
(c) Both (a) and (b) (d) None of them

13. Unconjugated bilirubin:

(a) Not excreted in urine (b) Excreted in urine
(c) Both (a) and (b) (d) None of them

14. Bilirubin in urine is tested by:

(a) Gmelin's test (b) Fouchet's test
(c) Sulphanilic acid (d) All of them

15. Aspartate transaminase (AST) is found in:

(a) Cytoplasm (b) Mitochondria
(c) Both (a) and (b) (d) None of them

16. Galactose tolerance is markedly elevated in:

(a) Cirrhosis (b) Infective hepatitis

(c) Both (a) and (b) (d) None of them

17. Albumin has a half life of:

(a) 20-25 days (b) 30-40 days

(c) 10-15 days (d) 0-10 days

18. Serum electrophoresis of proteins reveals:

(a) Increased albumin (b) Increased γ-globulin

(c) Decreased albumin (d) None of them

19. When the liver function is impaired, concentration of plasma clotting factors:

(a) Increased (b) Decreased

(c) Remains same (d) None of them

20. Half life of clotting factors is:

(a) 5-18 days (b) 5-36 hours

(c) 5-54 hours (d) 5-72 hours

21. Prothrombin time is prolonged due to the deficiency of:

(a) Vitamin K (b) Vitamin E

(c) Vitamin A (d) Vitamin C

22. Kidneys are responsible for the regulation of:

(a) Water (b) Electrolyte

(c) Acid-base balance (d) All of them

23. Kidneys reabsorb and retain several substances of bio-chemical importance:

(a) Glucose (b) Amino acid

(c) Both (a) and (b) (d) None of them

24. Erythropoietin, a peptide hormone stimulates:

(a) Hemoglobin synthesis (b) Erythrocyte formation

(c) Both (a) and (b) (d) None of them

25. The process of urine formation involves:

(a) Glomerular filtration (b) Tubular reabsorption

(c) Both (a) and (b) (d) None of them

26. Kidney function tests are:

(a) Glomerular function test (b) Tubular function test

(c) Urine examination (d) All of them

27. To assess renal function, following estimation will be useful:

(a) Blood urea (b) Serum creatinine

(c) Serum protein (d) All of them

28. Kidney functioning is assessed by routine examination of urine for:

(a) Volume (b) pH

(c) Abnormal constituents (d) All of them

29. The excretion of creatinine in urine is constant and not influenced by:

(a) Body metabolism (b) Dietary factors

(c) Either (a) or (b) (d) Neither (a) or (b)

30. The functions of stomach:

(a) Great churning ability (b) Elaborates HCl and pepsin

(c) Reservoir of ingested food stuffs (d) All of them

31. The test to assess gastric function:

(a) Insulin test meal (b) Pentagastrin stimulation test

(c) Augmented histamine test meal (d) All of them

32. Increased gastric HCl secretion is found in:

(a) Chronic duodenal ulcer (b) Gastric cell hyperplasia

(c) Excessive histamine production (d) All of them

33. A decrease in gastric HCl is observed in:

(a) Gastritis (b) Gastric carcinoma

(c) Pernicious anemia (d) All of them

34. Serum amylase and lipase activities are elevated in:

(a) Acute pancreatitis (b) Obstruction in intestine

(c) Obstruction in pancreatic duct (d) All of them

35. Pancreatitis may be extra pancreatic in origin as in:

(a) Acute appendicitis (b) Biliary obstruction

(c) Intrapancreatic (d) Either (a) or (b) or (c)

36. The enzyme carbonic anhydrase is of central importance in the renal regulation of pH, which occurs by:

(a) Excretion of H^+ ions (b) Reabsorption of bicarbonate

(c) Excretion of titratable acid (d) All of them

37. The weight of each kidney in grams is about:

(a) 90-130 (b) 120-170

(c) 100-110 (d) None of them

38. The daily normal total amount of urine contains the number of grams of solids:

(a) 35 (b) 50

(c) 60 (b) 90

39. The urinary excretion increases by the following substance having a diuretic action:

(a) Urea (b) Cellulose

(c) Glycerol (d) None of them

40. Decreased urine volume is seen in:

(a) Acute nephritis (b) Fever

(c) Diseases of heart (d) All of them

41. The chief pigment of urine:

(a) Coproporphyrin (b) Terochrome

(c) Urobilinogen (d) Uroerythrin

42. In liver disease the colour of urine may be:

(a) Green (b) Brown

(c) Deep yellow (d) All of them

43. The colour of urine is dark brown due to:

(a) Methemoglobin (b) Homogentisic acid

(c) Both (a) and (b) (d) None of them

44. A turbidity is developed in alkaline urine by the precipitation of:

(a) Calcium phosphate (b) Magnesium sulphate

(c) Both (a) and (b) (d) None of them

45. Strongly acid urine is pink due to precipitation of:

(a) Chloride salts (b) Ammonium salts

(c) Uric acid salt (d) None of them

46. The urine is acid in high protein intake due to the excess formation of:

(a) Sulphates (b) Phosphates

(c) Both (a) and (b) (d) None of them

47. Urea excretion is increased in:

(a) Fever (b) Diabetes

(c) Excess adrenocortical activity (d) None of them

48. In urine, output of high ammonia is in:

(a) Uncontrolled diabetes mellitus (b) Cirrhosis of liver

(c) Uremia (d) Nephritis

49. Creatine excretion is found in:

(a) Starvation (b) Infection

(c) Hyperthyroidism (d) All of them

50. Uric acid excretion is increased in:

(a) Leukemia (b) Severe liver disease

(c) Various stages of gout (d) All of them

51. The number of mg of amino acid nitrogen excreted in the urine of adults daily is about:

(a) 100-150 (b) 150-200

(c) 200-250 (d) None of them

52. Increased amount of amino acids is excreted in:

(a) Liver disease (b) Certain types of poisoning

(c) Both (a) and (b) (d) None of them

53. Proteinuria also results in the poisoning of renal tubules by heavy metals:

(a) Mercury (b) Arsenic

(c) Bismuth (d) All of them

54. Sodium and potassium excretion are controlled by the activity of:

(a) Adrenal medulla (b) Adrenal cortex

(c) Thyroid (d) None of them

55. The number of mg of protein present in normal urine cannot be detected by ordinary tests:

(a) 30-200 (b) 40-250

(c) 60-300 (d) None of them

56. Decrease in phosphate excretion is observed in:

(a) Hypoparathyroidism (b) Infectious diseases

(c) Both (a) and (b) (d) None of them

57. Phosphate excretion is increased in:

(a) Wasting diseases of nervous system (b) Osteomalacia

(c) Renal tubular rickets (d) All of them

58. The amino acid excreted in urine in cystinuria:

(a) Arginine (b) Cystine

(c) Lysine (d) All of them

59. In uremia, the concentration of urea and other non-protein nitrogenous constituents in plasma are:

(a) Increased (b) Decreased

(c) Remains same (d) None of them

60. Renal tubular acidosis is accompanied by excessive mobilization and urinary excretion of:

(a) Calcium (b) Potassium

(c) Both (a) and (b) (d) None of them

61. Radio-active scanning is useful for the detection of abnormalities in kidney's:

(a) Size (b) Shape

(c) Position (d) All of them

62. In case of normal renal function, excretion of water is:

(a) Less than 80 per cent (b) More then 80 per cent

(c) Both (a) and (b) (d) None of them

63. In case of impaired renal function, excretion of water is:

(a) More than 80 per cent (b) Less than 80 per cent

(c) Both (a) and (b) (d) None of them

64. Changes taking place in urine on storage are:

(a) Oxidation of urobilinogen to urobilin

(b) Rapid oxidation of ascorbic acid

(c) Action of micro-organisms on glucose

(d) All of them

65. The urine can be preserved by:

(a) Concentrated HCl (b) Formaldehyde

(c) Chloroform (d) All of them

66. The urine affected by bacteria is unsuitable for the determination of:

(a) pH (b) Urea

(c) Total nitrogen (d) All of them

67. Alkaline urine occurs as a result of retention of urine in bladder due to:

(a) Cystitis (b) Obstructive lesions

(c) Either (a) or (b) (d) Neither (a) or (b)

68. Alkaline urine is observed during:

(a) Metabolic alkalosis (b) Ingestion of sodium acetate

(c) Sodium carbonate (d) All of them

69. Under abnormal conditions, specific gravity of urine may be below normal due to:

(a) Inability to concentrate urine (b) Inability to excrete water

(c) Both (a) and (b) (d) None of them

70. In pathological urine, samples may contain organized elements like:

(a) Leucocytes (b) Erythrocytes

(c) Epithelial cells (d) All of them

71. In pathological urine, samples may contain unorganized elements like:

(a) Fat droplets (b) Crystals

(c) Pigments (d) All of them

72. The amount of urine produced per day by normal animal depends on:

(a) Climate (b) Diet

(c) Fluid intake (d) All of them

73. The condition of oligouria (less urine) is seen in:

(a) Chronic renal failure (b) Vomiting

(c) Diarrheoa (d) All of them

74. The condition of anuria (no urine) is seen in:

(a) Acute nephritis (b) Collapses

(c) Both (a) and (b) (d) None of them

75. Glycosuria occurs in:

(a) Diabetes mellitus
(b) Hyperthyroidism
(c) Hyperpituitarism
(d) All of them

76. When glucose in urine is tested by Benedict's test, the colour of precipitate obtained is:

(a) Red
(b) Yellow
(c) Green
(d) Either (a) or (b) or (c)

77. Kidneys excrete albumin in renal albuminuria which shows:

(a) Altered blood pressure
(b) Altered kidney structure
(c) Both (a) and (b)
(d) None of them

78. A mild albuminuria may occur during:

(a) Infectious disease
(b) Violent exercise
(c) Both (a) and (b)
(d) None of them

79. In Heller's test for proteins in urine, a white ring is formed at the junction due to:

(a) Precipitation of proteins
(b) Coagulation of proteins
(c) Sedimentation of proteins
(d) None of them

80. Ketosis occurs during:

(a) Fasting
(b) Carbohydrate deprivation
(c) Either (a) or (b)
(d) Neither (a) or (b)

81. Ketosis occurs in:

(a) Fever
(b) Pregnancy
(c) Malnutrition
(d) All of them

82. In Hay's test for bile salts in urine, sulphur powder settles down at the bottom due to the reason:

(a) Bile salts lower surface tension
(b) Bile salts increase surface tension
(c) Both (a) and (b)
(d) None of them

83. Hemoglobinuria occurs in:

(a) Yellow fever
(b) Extensive burns
(c) Hemolytic anemia
(d) All of them

84. Hematuria occurs in:

(a) Acute glomerular nephritis (b) Stones in urinary tract
(c) Both (a) and (b) (d) None of them

85. In disease condition, the chemical composition of blood is influenced by the factors:

(a) Physical (b) Metabolic
(c) Both (a) and (b) (d) None of them

86. Physical factors include:

(a) Accumulation of nitrogenous waste products (nephritis)
(b) Increased transaminase activity of serum
(c) Hypercholestermia
(d) All of them

87. The functions of body in health and disease conditions are ascertained by determining concentration of various constituents of blood under the condition:

(a) Normal (b) Physiological
(c) Pathological (d) All of them

88. If blood is clotted for a longer period, more:

(a) The clot retracts (b) Serum obtained
(c) Both (a) and (b) (d) None of them

89. Excess of anticoagulant should be avoided because:

(a) pH of blood is shifted
(b) Precipitation of protein interfered
(c) Rapid loss of blood glucose
(d) All of them

90. The presence of protein in blood interferes with:

(a) Analysis of compounds containing amino nitrogen
(b) Analysis involving oxidation or reduction of metal ions
(c) Both (a) and (b)
(d) None of them

91. Sodium fluoride is used as an anticoagulant for blood glucose due to the reason:

(a) Enzymatic breakdown to lactic acid

(b) Disappearance of glucose on standing

(c) Both (a) and (b)

(d) None of them

92. For glucose estimation, Folin-Wu tube is used, the constricted neck of which:

(a) Decreases surface exposed to atmosphere

(b) Prevents oxidation of cuprous ions to cupric ions

(c) Both (a) and (b)

(d) None of them

93. Albumin level decreases in:

(a) Severe burns
(b) Nephritis
(c) Chronic liver disease
(d) All of them

94. Globulin level increases in:

(a) Chronic infection
(b) Multiple myeloma
(c) Advanced liver disease
(b) All of them

95. Hypercholestermia is seen in:

(a) Nephrosis
(b) Myxoedema
(c) Obstructive Jaundice
(d) All of them

96. Hypocholestermia is seen in:

(a) Anemia
(b) Hemolytic jaundice
(c) Both (a) and (b)
(d) None of them

97. Conjugated bilirubin is increased in:

(a) Obstructive jaundice
(b) Hemolytic jaundice
(c) Hepatic jaundice
(d) None of them

98. Higher value of blood urea can be seen in:

(a) Chronic intestinal obstruction
(b) Ulcerative colitis
(c) Severe vomiting
(d) All of them

99. Increased level of uric acid is found in:

(a) Gout
(b) Renal failure
(c) Megaloblastic anemia
(d) All of them

100. Increased plasma chloride level is seen in:

(a) Alkalosis (b) Acidosis
(c) Hydremia (d) None of them

101. The causes of hyperkalemia are:

(a) Hemolysis (b) Leucocytosis
(c) Thrombocytosis (d) All of them

102. Decreased magnesium level of blood serum is found in:

(a) Chronic nephritis (b) Oxalate poisoning
(c) Hypomagnesemia tetany (d) None of them

103. The total serum calcium may be affected by deficient intestinal absorption of calcium by altered:

(a) Bone metabolism (b) Renal excretion
(c) Plasma protein (d) All of them

104. In jaundice excessive hemolysis could be due to:

(a) Congenital abnormality of RBC (b) Abnormal hemoglobin
(c) Enzyme defects (d) All of them

105. In early renal disease or failure, sensitive is:

(a) Creatinine (b) BUN
(c) Either (a) or (b) (d) Neither (a) or (b)

106. Diabetes mellitus in dog, cat, cow and sheep may arise due to:

(a) Acute pancreatic necrosis (b) Pituitary neoplasms
(c) Adrenal hyperplasia (d) All of them

107. The absorption of glucose is affected by:

(a) Gastrointestinal acidity (b) Digestive enzymes
(c) Disease (d) All of them

108. The process of exclusion in closely related diseases is known as:

(a) Test therapy diagnosis (b) Clinical diagnosis
(c) Laboratory diagnosis (d) Differential diagnosis

109. Coagulation time increases in:

(a) Warferian poisoning (b) Hemophilia
(c) Both (a) and (b) (d) None of them

110. Canines have more ________ than lymphocytes:

(a) Monocytes (b) Eosinophils

(c) Neutrophils (d) Basophils

111. Increased erythrocyte sedimentation rate is an indication of:

(a) Malignancy (b) Nephritis

(c) Tuberculosis (d) All of them

112. If blood is present in feces, it is known as:

(a) Hematuria (b) Melena

(c) Dysentry (d) All of them

113. Red colour urine is observed in:

(a) Hematuria (b) Phenothiazine toxicity

(c) Both (a) and (b) (d) None of them

114. Proteinuria may occur in:

(a) Glomerular-nephritis (b) Pyelonephritis

(c) Both (a) and (b) (d) None of them

115. Myoglobulin in urine is detected in:

(a) Strangles (b) Glanders

(c) Azoturia (d) Equine infectious anemia

116. Number of pus cells increase in urine due to:

(a) Pyelonephritis (b) Pasteurellosis

(c) Tuberculosis (d) Brucellosis

117. Presence of more than _____ chloride content is considered abnormal:

(a) 1.0% (b) 0.1%

(c) 0.001% (d) 0.01%

118. Glucose level of synovial fluid ____ in joint diseases:

(a) Increases (b) Decreases

(c) Remains same (d) None of them

119. In joint diseases, the level of alkaline phosphatase in synovial fluid:

(a) Increases (b) Decreases

(c) Remains same (d) None of them

120. In inflammatory conditions of joints, the synovial fluid clots within:

(a) 2 hrs (b) 3 hrs

(c) 5 hrs (d) None of them

121. Specific gravity of synovial fluid more than _______ is indicative of arthritis:

(a) 1.020 (b) 1.010

(c) 1.030 (d) 1.015

122. Protein content of synovial fluid increases more than ______ g/100ml in joint diseases of cattle:

(a) 1.0 (b) 2.0

(c) 3.0 (d) 6.0

123. Increased level of creatine kinase in cerebrospinal fluid is considered ______ sign of prognosis:

(a) Favourable (b) Good

(c) Poor (d) None of them

124. Elevation of AST and ALT in cerebrospinal fluid is an indication of:

(a) Infectious canine hepatitis (b) Canine parvoviral infection

(c) Rabies (d) Canine distemper

125. In cerebrospinal fluid glucose concentration is___ of blood glucose concentration:

(a) 50-60 % (b) 60-70 %

(c) 70-80% (d) 80-90%

126. Cerebrospinal fluid may become turbid in:

(a) Purpulent encephalomyelitis (b) Encephalomalacia

(c) Meningioencephalitis (d) Brain tumors

127. Increased serum AST may be an indication of hepatic cell necrosis in:

(a) Dog (b) Cat

(c) Primates (d) All of them

128. Increased activity of AST in horses is seen in:

(a) Septicemia (b) Intestinal complications

(c) Hepatitis (d) All of them

129. Increased enzyme concentrations are a measure of:

(a) Organ damage (b) Decreased organ function

(c) Both (a) and (b) (d) None of them

130. Increase of a particular enzyme depends on its:

(a) Rate of release (b) Rate of production

(c) Rate of clearance (d) All of them

131. Liver function tests based on the changes in plasma proteins (disturbances in protein metabolism):

(a) Flocculation test

(b) Amino acids in blood and urine

(c) Determination of total serum protein and A/G ratio

(d) All of them

132. Liver is an important site for cholesterol:

(a) Biosynthesis (b) Esterification

(c) Oxidation (d) All of them

133. Smaller sized stones are found in:

(a) Kidney (b) Renal pelvis

(c) Both (a) and (b) (d) Urinary bladder

134. Urinary calculi are:

(a) Simple calculi (b) Mixed calculi

(c) Foreign body calculi (d) All of them

135. More than 90% stones contain the following:

(a) Uric acid (b) Urates

(c) Oxalates (d) All of them

136. Uric acid crystals dissolve in:

(a) Sodium hydroxide (b) Acetic acid

(c) Hydrochloric acid (d) None of them

137. Calcium oxalate may be found in the deposits from:

(a) Acidic urine (b) Alkaline urine

(c) Both (a) and (b) (d) None of them

138. Factors causing stone formation:

(a) Stagnation of urine (b) Presence of infection

(c) Both (a) and (b) (d) None of them

139. Kidney function tests help in:

(a) Locating the site of impairment of renal function

(b) Providing information concerning normal functioning of kidney cells

(c) Both (a) and (b)

(d) None of them

140. In renal diseases, kidney becomes unable to:

(a) Dilute the urine

(b) Concentrate the urine

(c) Both (a) and (b)

(d) None of them

141. Freshly passed urine has aromatic smell due to:

(a) Volatile organic acids

(b) Bacterial hydrolysis of urea to ammonia

(c) Either (a) or (b)

(d) Neither (a) or (b)

142. Kidney functions are regulated by the hormone:

(a) Vasopressin

(b) Parathormone

(c) Aldosterone

(d) All of them

143. Main functions of kidney are:

(a) Regulation of H^+ concentration of blood

(b) Maintenance of osmotic pressure of blood

(c) Regulation of arterial blood pressure

(d) All of them

144. Pathological aminoaciduria is due to:

(a) Increased concentration of amino acid

(b) Defective renal tubular reabosrption

(c) Both (a) and (b)

(d) None of them

145. The amount of potassium in urine increases with:

(a) Increase in alkalosis

(b) Decrease in alkalosis

(c) Increase in acidosis

(d) None of them

146. Aldosterone increases the reabsorption of:

(a) Na^+ ions

(b) K^+ ions

(c) Either (a) or (b)

(d) Neither (a) or (b)

147. In urine the excretion of sodium per day is:

(a) 2-4 g
(b) 3-5 g
(c) 4-6 g
(d) 7-8 g

148. Repeated analysis of serum creatinine in kidney disorders helps in:

(a) Diagnosis
(b) Prognosis
(c) Both (a) and (b)
(d) None of them

149. The level of globulin content increases in:

(a) Bacterial
(b) Viral
(c) Parasitic infection
(d) All of them

150. The serum protein measurement is indicated in:

(a) Liver disease
(b) Immunosuppression
(c) Chronic wasting diseases
(d) All of them

Answer Key

1	(c)	26	(d)	51	(b)	76	(d)
2	(d)	27	(d)	52	(c)	77	(c)
3	(d)	28	(d)	53	(d)	78	(c)
4	(d)	29	(c)	54	(b)	79	(a)
5	(d)	30	(d)	55	(a)	80	(c)
6	(c)	31	(d)	56	(c)	81	(d)
7	(d)	32	(d)	57	(d)	82	(a)
8	(d)	33	(d)	58	(d)	83	(d)
9	(c)	34	(d)	59	(a)	84	(c)
10	(b)	35	(d)	60	(c)	85	(c)
11	(c)	36	(d)	61	(d)	86	(d)
12	(a)	37	(b)	62	(b)	87	(d)
13	(a)	38	(c)	63	(b)	88	(c)
14	(d)	39	(a)	64	(d)	89	(d)
15	(c)	40	(d)	65	(d)	90	(c)
16	(c)	41	(b)	66	(d)	91	(c)
17	(a)	42	(d)	67	(c)	92	(c)
18	(a)	43	(c)	68	(d)	93	(d)
19	(b)	44	(a)	69	(c)	94	(d)
20	(d)	45	(c)	70	(d)	95	(d)
21	(a)	46	(c)	71	(d)	96	(c)
22	(d)	47	(d)	72	(d)	97	(a)
23	(c)	48	(a)	73	(d)	98	(d)
24	(c)	49	(d)	74	(c)	99	(a)
25	(c)	50	(d)	75	(d)	100	(a)

101	(d)	114	(c)	127	(d)	140	(c)
102	(c)	115	(c)	128	(d)	141	(a)
103	(d)	116	(a)	129	(a)	142	(d)
104	(d)	117	(b)	130	(d)	143	(d)
105	(d)	118	(a)	131	(d)	144	(c)
106	(d)	119	(b)	132	(d)	145	(a)
107	(d)	120	(b)	133	(c)	146	(a)
108	(d)	121	(b)	134	(d)	147	(b)
109	(c)	122	(a)	135	(d)	148	(c)
110	(c)	123	(c)	136	(a)	149	(d)
111	(d)	124	(d)	137	(c)	150	(d)
112	(b)	125	(b)	138	(c)		
113	(c)	126	(a)	139	(c)		

Chapter 21

Animal Biotechnology

1. **The optimum temperature of Taq DNA polymerase is:**
   (a) 54°C (b) 94°C
   (c) 72°C (d) 60°C
2. **Microbes used in the manufacture of cheese by fermentation:**
   (a) Lactobacillus (b) *E.coli*
   (c) Lamdaphage (d) None of the above
3. **The primer used in PCR is 10-20 bases in length which is complimentary to the templates at its:**
   (a) 5' end (b) 3' end
   (c) Both (a) and (b) (d) None of the above
4. **The vector DNA used for constructing a genomic library is:**
   (a) Plasmid (b) Bacteriophage
   (c) Cosmid (d) None of the above
5. **Double chained DNA strand is made radioactive in both its chains. It is allowed to replicate twice in non-radioactive medium. The result would be:**
   (a) All strands have radioactivity
   (b) Half the strands have radioactivity
   (c) Three strands have radioactivity
   (d) Radioactivity is absent in all the strands

6. **The most common plasmid vector used in genetic engineering is:**
   (a) PBR 328 (b) PBR 325
   (c) PBR 330 (d) PBR 322
7. **In PCR primers bind to strand at:**
   (a) 10-30°C (b) 30-60°C
   (c) 60-80°C (d) 80-100°C
8. **Recombinant DNA can be introduced into the bacterial cell in presence of:**
   (a) Sodium phosphate (b) Potassium phosphate
   (c) Calcium phosphate (d) Magnesium phosphate
9. **The arm required for recognition of amino acid is present in:**
   (a) mRNA (b) tRNA
   (c) rRNA (d) SnRNA
10. **The culture medium used to sort out the hybridoma cells from others is:**
    (a) HAT (b) RAT
    (c) CAT (d) SAT
11. **Expression vectors differ from a cloning vector in having:**
    (a) An origin of replication (b) Suitable marker genes
    (c) Unique restriction sites (d) Control elements
12. **Which is not a method of Identification of protein:**
    (a) PCR (b) Mass spcctrometry
    (c) NMR (d) X-ray crystallography
13. **Linear DNA molecules with several restriction enzyme sites are:**
    (a) Bacteriophages (b) Plasmids
    (c) Cosmids (d) All of the above
14. **Melting of target DNA is known as:**
    (a) Denaturation (b) Annealing
    (c) Polymerization (d) None of them
15. **Tumor marker can be detected by:**
    (a) Immuno histochemistry (b) Immunofluorescence
    (c) Agglutinaion (d) Complement fixation test

16. In gel electrophoresis we use:
(a) Agar agar powder
(b) Polyacrylamide gel
(c) Sodium chloride
(d) Blood agar

17. The event of entering the plasmid containing DNA fragment into a bacterial cell in known as:
(a) Transformation
(b) Transfection
(c) Polymerization
(d) Transcription

18. Monoclonal antibodies are used to:
(a) Detect allergies
(b) Diagnose viral diseases
(c) Detect certain types of cancers
(d) All of the above

19. Conversion of cultured cells into cancerous cells is known as:
(a) Transformation
(b) Translation
(c) Both (a) and (b)
(d) None of them

20. Southern blotting is hybridization of:
(a) DNA
(b) RNA
(c) Protein
(d) None of them

21. Readily available and less expensive sera for culture media are:
(a) Foetal bovine
(b) Bovine calf serum
(c) Both (a) and (b)
(d) None of them

22. Polyacrylamide gel electrophoresis is used for separating:
(a) RNA
(b) Protein
(c) Both (a) and (b)
(d) None of them

23. Western blotting technique is used for finding:
(a) Protein
(b) DNA
(c) RNA
(d) All of them

24. Prostaglandin is given_____hrs after initiation of FSH treatment in cattle in oestrus synchronization and superovulation protocol of MOET:
(a) 48 hrs
(b) 72 hrs
(c) 24 hrs
(d) 36 hrs

25. Basic technique used for synchronization of oestrus:
(a) Prolongation of luteal phase
(b) Induction of luteolysis/ shortening
(c) Both (a) and (b)
(d) None of the above

26. Rumen digestion can be improved by:

(a) Inclusion of probiotic
(b) Chelated minerals
(c) Transfer of rumen microbes
(d) All of the above organism

27. Vaccines used to differentiate between infected animals are known as:

(a) Malaria vaccine
(b) Marker vaccine
(c) Either (a) or (b)
(d) Neither (a) or (b)

28. Which is not an embryo sexing technique:

(a) Detection of X-chromatin mass
(b) Use of Y- specific DNA probe
(c) Detection of H-Y antigen
(d) Use of particle gun

29. Which is not a method of gene transfer:

(a) Chromosome analysis
(b) Use of virus
(c) Fusion of cells
(d) All of them

30. Oocyte can be collected from large animals by:

(a) Slaughter house ovaries
(b) Trans-vaginal ultra sound guided ovum pickup technique
(c) Both (a) and (b)
(d) None of them

31. Which of the following is not a non-invasive method of sexing of embryo:

(a) H-Y antigen detection
(b) Measurement of X-linked enzyme activity
(c) Both (a) and (b)
(d) Karyotyping

32. Which of the following is non-invasive advanced technique in animal reproduction:

(a) Ultrasonography
(b) Aminocentesis
(c) Leproscopy
(d) Endometrial biopsy

33. Vaccinia virus is used as a vector as it has:

(a) Small genome
(b) Relatively difficult to insert new genome
(c) It can not express high level of new antigen
(d) Recombinant proteins undergo appropriate processing steps within vaccinia

34. Green fluorescent proteins are used to monitor the activity of:

(a) Transcription (b) Translation
(c) Both (a) and (b) (d) None of them

35. Genetic diseases impending protein maturation are:

(a) Scrapie (b) Alzheimer's disease
(c) Mad cow disease (d) None of them

36. Streptomycin prevents proper chain initiation and thereby causes cell death at:

(a) Higher concentration (b) Lower concentration
(c) Both (a) and (b) (d) None of them

37. In prokaryotes and eukaryotes fundamental principles of transcription are:

(a) Similar (b) Dissimilar
(c) Both (a) and (b) (d) None of them

38. A number of host properties are specified by plasmids like:

(a) Nitrogen fixation (b) Pollutant degradation
(c) Heavy metal resistance (d) All of them

39. Plasmids are DNA molecules, which are:

(a) Extra chromosomal (b) Self replicating
(c) Double stranded (d) All of them

40. Recombinant DNA technology helps in understanding the molecular basis of diseases like:

(a) Sickle cell anemia (b) Thalassemias
(c) Both (a) and (b) (d) None of them

41. Recombinant DNA technology applies to the production of compounds like:

(a) Insulin (b) Blood clotting factor
(c) Vaccines (d) All of them

42. The shuttle vector is:

(a) Stable (b) Non-pathogenic
(c) Non-stress inducing (d) All of them

43. Terminator sequence provides signal for:

(a) Termination of transcription (b) Initiation of transcription
(c) Both (a) and (b) (d) None of them

44. Vector has got the property of:

(a) Autonomous replication (b) Specific nucleotide sequence
(c) Gene for identification (d) All of them

45. DNA fragments length, which cosmids can accept is:

(a) 25-50kb (b) 10-20kb
(c) 6-10kb (d) None of them

46. DNA fragments length, which plasmids can accept :

(a) 6-10kb (b) 10-20kb
(c) 25-50kb (d) All of them

47. DNA fragments length, which bacteriophages can accept:

(a) 10-20kb (b) 25-50kb
(c) 6-10kb (d) None of them

48. Following can be used for the preparation of chimeric DNA:

(a) A fragment of target DNA (b) A fragment of vector DNA
(c) Both (a) and (b) (d) None of them

49. By polymerase chain reaction, millions of copies of DNA fragments can be synthesized in:

(a) Few hours (b) Few minutes
(c) Few seconds (d) None of them

50. Polymerase chain reaction is suited where the quantity of biological specimen available is:

(a) Very low (b) Very high
(c) Neither (a) or (b) (d) Both (a) and (b)

51. Taq polymerase survives for 1-2 minutes at:

(a) 95°C (b) 80°C
(c) 70°C (d) 60°C

52. Taq polymerase has half life at 95°C:

(a) More than 2 hours (b) Less than 2 hours
(c) More than 4 hours (d) None of them

53. DNA is heat denatured for 15 seconds at:

(a) 95°C (b) 90°C
(c) 85°C (d) None of them

54. Polymerase chain reaction employes the enzyme:

(a) Taq polymerase (b) Vent polymerase
(c) Both (a) and (b) (d) None of them

55. After the completion of one cycle of polymerase chain reaction, number of strands produced are:

(a) 4 (b) 8
(c) 16 (d) 32

56. In polymerase chain reaction, 20 cycles will produce about:

(a) One million copies of DNA (b) One billion copies of DNA
(c) Two million copies of DNA (d) None of them

57. The following disease can be detected by using polymerase chain reaction:

(a) Sickle cell anemia (b) Muscular dystrophy
(c) Phenyl ketonuria (d) All of them

58. DNA finger printing is used in forensic science to search:

(a) Criminals (b) Rapists
(c) Both (a) and (b) (d) None of them

59. DNA finger printing can identify:

(a) Burnt dead body (b) Unidentifiable dead body
(c) Both (a) and (b) (d) None of them

60. The biological samples required for DNA profiling are:

(a) Blood stain (b) Skin cells
(c) Piece of hair with root (d) All of them

61. Genome sequencing is done to know:

(a) Total number of all genes
(b) Relationship between genes
(c) Genetic information about the organism
(d) All of them

62. Structural genomics deals with:

(a) DNA sequencing

(b) Sequence assembly

(c) Sequence organisms and management

(d) All of them

63. Functional genomics deals with the study of function of:

(a) All gene sequences (b) Gene sequence expression

(c) Both (a) and (b) (d) None of them

64. Proteomics is the proteome's:

(a) Identification (b) Analysis

(c) Characterization (d) All of them

65. DNA has important role in the cell:

(a) Replication (b) Expression

(c) Both (a) and (b) (d) None of them

66. Gene expression refers to protein synthesis through:

(a) Transcription (b) Translation

(c) Both (a) and (b) (d) None of them

67. Central dogma is the transfer of information from DNA to:

(a) Protein (b) RNA

(c) Either of the two (d) Neither of the two

68. Gene expression of prokaryotes is controlled at the stage:

(a) Transcription (b) Translation

(c) Both (a) and (b) (d) None of them

69. An operon consists of:

(a) Repressor (b) Promoter

(c) Structural gene (d) All of them

70. Reverse transcriptase is very useful in the synthesis of:

(a) cDNA (b) cDNA clone bank

(c) Both (a) and (b) (d) None of them

71. A gene library is the collection of different DNA sequences each has been cloned into a vector for ease of:

(a) Purification (b) Storage

(c) Analysis (d) All of them

72. Genomic DNA is fragmented by:

(a) Restriction enzyme digestion (b) Physical shearing
(c) Both (a) and (b) (d) None of them

73. Genomic library represents an organism's:

(a) Complete genome (b) Complete proteome
(c) Either of the two (d) Neither of the two

74. Genomic DNA of eukaryotes contains:

(a) Introns (b) Regulatory regions
(c) Repetitive sequences (d) All of them

75. The cDNA library represents the DNA of:

(a) Eukaryotic organisms (b) Prokaryotic organisms
(c) Either of the two (d) Neither of the two

76. Disease diagnosis can be done by genetic engineering technique:

(a) DNA probe (b) Monoclonal antibodies
(c) Antenatal diagnosis (d) All of them

77. Monoclonal antibodies are used in the diagnosis of:

(a) Cancer (b) Pregnancy
(c) Viral diseases (d) All of them

78. Somatic gene therapy holds promise for the disorder:

(a) Cancer (b) Neurological disorder
(c) Heart disease (d) All of them

79. The success of gene therapy depends on:

(a) Gene delivery mechanism (b) Choice of target tissue
(c) Both (a) and (b) (d) None of them

80. The circulating antigens in the blood can be assayed by using:

(a) ELISA (b) RIA
(c) Either of the two (d) Neither of the two

81. By using ELISA, following can be tested:

(a) Hepatitis (b) HIV
(c) Typhoid (d) All of them

82. Embryo transfer method can not be used widely due to:

(a) High cost (b) Technical difficulty

(c) Limited supply of embryo (d) All of them

83. The time of ovulation in cow and horse is:

(a) 21 days (b) 16 days

(c) 10 days (d) None of them

84. The time of ovulation in sheep and goat is:

(a) 16 days (b) 21 days

(c) 10 days (d) None of them

85. In well managed cattles, number of eggs superovulated depends on:

(a) Health (b) Nutrition

(c) Breed (d) All of them

86. The percentage of pregnancy achieved by embryo transfer method in cattle is:

(a) 30-40 (b) 40-50

(c) 50-60 (d) None of them

87. Through normal reproduction an animal in her life produces:

(a) 2-3 offsprings (b) 3-4 offsprings

(c) 4-5 offsprings (d) None of them

88. Transgenic animals can be used as bioreactors for large scale production of:

(a) Hormones (b) Interferons

(c) Proteins (d) All of them

89. The transected cultural mammalian cells have been used for the diagnostic of:

(a) Oncogens (b) Gene therapy

(c) Both (a) and (b) (d) None of them

90. Genetic markers can be used to detect the presence of specific:

(a) Genotype (b) Phenotype

(c) Either of the two (d) Neither of the two

91. Chromosomal study in cytology is termed as:

(a) Exfoliative cytology (b) Cytogenetics

(c) Cytochemistry (d) None of them

92. PCR inhibitors include:

(a) Heparin
(b) Proteinasek
(c) Porphyrin
(d) All of them

93. Confirmation of PCR products is done through:

(a) Nested PCR
(b) Southern blotting
(c) Both (a) and (b)
(d) None of them

94. Complementary DNA is formed from_____ for PCR:

(a) RNA
(b) Protein
(c) Carbohydrate
(d) Fat

95. The hybridized nucleic acid on nitrocellulose membrane are exposed to X-ray for _____ for its characterization:

(a) Microscopy
(b) Biopsy
(c) Autoradiography
(d) Cytology

96. *In situ* hybridization technique is more useful in diagnosis of such viruses which are:

(a) Cultivable
(b) Non-cultivable
(c) Both (a) and (b)
(d) None of them

97. Amplification of nucleic acid from small amount in clinical sample is known as:

(a) ELISA
(b) SDS-PAGE
(c) DIA
(d) PCR

98. Blood agar is a ______ media:

(a) Simple
(b) Enriched
(c) Selective
(d) None of them

99. Agglutination test can be carried out when antigen is in ____ form:

(a) Soluble
(b) Particulate
(c) Both (a) and (b)
(d) None of them

100. Continuous cell lines used for virus cultures can survive for _____ passage:

(a) 5
(b) 10
(c) 20
(d) Indefinite

101. Agar gel precipitation test was first developed by:

(a) Widal
(b) Hirst
(c) Papanicolaou
(d) Ochterlony

102. Polymerase chain reaction was developed by:

(a) Kary Mullis
(b) Chand
(c) Albert Coons
(d) None of them

103. Genomic DNA is subjected to agarose gel electrophoresis to check the:

(a) Quality
(b) Purity
(c) Concentration
(d) All of them

104. Following Sanger's method of DNA sequencing, when DNA fragments are electrophoresed, smaller fragments move towards:

(a) Anode
(b) Cathode
(c) Both (a) and (b)
(d) None of them

105. On the basis of increasing order of fragment size (DNA), the lanes are read from:

(a) Anodic end to cathodic end
(b) Cathodic end to anodic end
(c) Either (a) or (b)
(d) Neither (a) or (b)

106. Following Sanger's method of DNA sequencing, when DNA fragments are electrophoresed, larger fragments move towards:

(a) Cathode
(b) Anode
(c) Either (a) or (b)
(d) Neither (a) or (b)

107. Plasmids are found in:

(a) Bacteria
(b) Cyanobacteria
(c) Fungi
(d) All of them

108. The forms of plasmid are:

(a) Super-coiled
(b) Relaxed
(c) Linear
(d) All of them

109. In the alkaline lysis method of plasmid isolation, cells are lysed using:

(a) SDS detergent
(b) EDTA
(c) Both (a) and (b)
(d) None of them

110. In alkaline lysis method for plasmid isolation, SDS:

(a) Removes lipid molecules
(b) Disrupts cell membrane
(c) Denatures bacterial proteins
(d) All of them

111. The proteins, DNA and RNA have electric charges which depend on:

(a) Molecule to molecule
(b) Conditions of medium
(c) Both (a) and (b)
(d) None of them

112. Due to the difference in amino acid composition, proteins have a unique:

(a) Mass (b) Charge

(c) Both (a) and (b) (d) None of them

113. SDS-PAGE name due to the reason, the proteins are treated first with:

(a) Sodium dodecyl sulphate (SDS) before the start

(b) During the course of electrophoresis (PAGE)

(c) Both (a) and (b)

(d) None of them

114. SDS-PAGE is normally used due to:

(a) Gel suppresses conventional current (b) Gel acts as molecular sieve

(c) Both (a) and (b) (d) None of them

115. Lower concentration of agarose gel is required for the separation of:

(a) DNA (b) RNA

(c) Plasmids (d) All of them

116. Agar gel have pore size:

(a) 100-300nm (b) 100-200nm

(c) 100-150nm (d) None of them

117. Embryo biopsy is very necessary in breeding to detect:

(a) Sex (b) Genetic diseases

(c) Both (a) and (b) (d) None of them

118. Surrogate mothers do not contribute any thing in terms of genetic makeup since the same comes from:

(a) Semen from artificial insemination (b) Egg of donor mother

(c) Both (a) and (b) (d) None of them

119. *In vitro* fertilization of eggs is carried out in micro droplets of culture medium, which should be supplemented with:

(a) Penicillamine (b) Hypotaurin

(c) Epinephrine (d) All of them

120. Before birth about 80 per cent genes play a key role in:

(a) Differentiation of foetuses (b) Development of foetuses

(c) Both (a) and (b) (d) None of them

121. For embryo cloning, technique used:

(a) Nuclear transplantation (b) Embryonic stem cells

(c) Both (a) and (b) (d) None of them

122. Nuclear transplantation experiment on embryonic cells of frog was carried out for the first time in 1955 by:

(a) Robert Briggs (b) Tom King

(c) Both (a) and (b) (d) None of them

123. The cloned animal produced via nuclear transplantation technique will be:

(a) Not capable of restoring fertility (b) Capable of restoring fertility

(c) Either (a) or (b) (d) Neither (a) or (b)

124. Embryonic stem (ES) cells are isolated:

(a) From inner cell mass of early embryo

(b) Without injecting transforming agent

(c) Either (a) or (b)

(d) None of them

125. Embryonic stem cells can be induced to generate:

(a) Muscle cells (b) Nerve cells

(c) Liver cells (d) All of them

126. Method of transfer of gene into animals is used to study the structure and function of genes through:

(a) Molecular markers (b) Genome mapping

(c) Both (a) and (b) (d) None of them

127. Marker genes are used to select the cells in which gene has been transferred at targeted site is achieved by:

(a) Polymerase chain reaction (PCR)

(b) Hypoxanthine phosphoribosyl transferase (HPRT)

(c) Both (a) and (b)

(d) None of them

128. Apoptosis results in:

(a) Loss of membrane integrity (b) Swelling of the cells

(c) Disrupture of the cells (b) All of them

129. The purpose of production of transgenic animals has been to produce:

(a) More protein in milk and meat (b) Disease resistance

(c) Good quality wool (d) All of them

130. Applications of molecular genetics in animals are:

(a) Breeding selective traits into livestock (b) Animal cell culture

(c) Production of transgenic animals (d) All of them

131. Molecular markers are:

(a) Hybridization based markers (b) PCR based markers

(c) Both (a) and (b) (d) None of them

132. Hybridization can also be carried out with the probes for different families of hypervariable repetitive DNA sequences like:

(a) Variable number of tandem repeats (b) Simple repeats

(c) Microsatellite (d) All of them

133. Molecular markers are:

(a) Distributed on genome

(b) Multiallelic

(c) Following typical mendalian inheritance

(d) All of them

134. For genetic analysis, molecular markers are advantageous in the sense, DNA can be:

(a) Isolated easily from blood and tissue

(b) Stored for a longer period

(c) Analyzed at an early age/embryonic stage

(d) All of them

135. By comparing a wide variety of genomes, following can be studied:

(a) Nature of horizontal gene transfer (b) Microbial evaluation

(c) Both (a) and (b) (d) None of them

136. The objectives of proteomics are:

(a) Characterization of post transcriptional modification in protein

(b) Preparation of 3D map of a cell indicating the exact location of protein

(c) Both (a) and (b)

(d) None of them

137. Areas of proteomics are:

(a) Protein expression
(b) Protein structure
(c) Protein-Protein interaction
(d) All of them

138. Interferon is used to cure viral diseases like:

(a) Hepatitis
(b) Common cold
(c) Both (a) and (b)
(d) All of them

139. In man the interferons are:

(a) Alpha interferon
(b) β- interferon
(c) γ- interferon
(d) All of them

140. Vaccines synthesized biologically, through genetic engineering:

(a) Vaccines for hepatitis B virus
(b) Vaccines for rabies virus
(c) Vaccines for polio virus
(d) All of them

141. Thalassaemia genes is a condition in which:

(a) α and β globin chain synthesis reduced
(b) Occurrence of hemolytic anemia
(c) Spleen enlargement
(d) All of them

142. Polymorphism observed at DNA sequence level has been playing a major role in human genetics for:

(a) Gene mapping
(b) Pre and post-natal diagnosis of diseases
(c) Anthropological and molecular evaluation studies
(d) All of them

143. Short range/immediate application of molecular markers are:

(a) Parentage determination
(b) Identification of disease carrier
(c) Sex determination
(d) All of them

144. Transgenesis has made possible to alter the:

(a) Structure of gene
(b) Function of gene
(c) Both (a) and (b)
(d) None of them

145. Molecular markers serve as a potential tool to geneticists and breeders for:

(a) Evaluating the existing germ plasm
(b) Manipulating it to create animals of desired traits
(c) Both (a) and (b)
(d) None of them

146. DNA microarray technology is useful in:

(a) Identification of tissue specific genes
(b) Discovery of drugs
(c) Variation in the cell cycle
(d) All of them

147. To study completely sequenced genomics, which one is to be analyzed:

(a) Nucleic acids (b) Proteins
(c) Both (a) and (b) (d) None of them

148. In order to understand genome organization and working of a living cell, the following information must be integrated:

(a) Variation in mRNA and protein levels (b) DNA and protein sequences
(c) Protein interaction (d) All of them

149. Success of gene therapy depends on the development of better gene transfer vectors for:

(a) Long term expression of foreign gene
(b) Better understanding of gene physiology
(c) Both (a) and (b)
(d) None of them

150. To initiate gene therapy, functional studies should be focused on:

(a) Design of newer vectors for gene delivery
(b) Targeting to specific tissues and cells
(c) Design of appropriate animal models
(d) All of them

151. Biotechnology is the integrated use of biochemistry, microbiology and engineering sciences in order to achieve technological application of the capability of:

(a) Micro-organism (b) Cultured tissue
(c) Tissue (d) All of them

152. Modern biotechnology embraces all the methods of genetic modification by:

(a) Recombinant DNA (b) Cell fusion technology

(c) Both (a) and (b) (d) None of them

153. Bio-informatics may be defined as application of information science to increase the understanding of:

(a) Biology (b) Biochemistry

(c) Biological data (d) All of them

154. Different types of genes of its known function have been made available by the construction of:

(a) Gene bank (b) DNA clone bank

(c) Both (a) and (b) (d) None of them

155. Bio diversity may be defined as the inherent and externally imposed variability within and among the living organisms present in:

(a) Terrestria (b) Marine

(c) Other ecosystem (d) All of them

156. Genes are functional entities of all organisms, because they determine:

(a) Physical features of organism

(b) Biological features of organisms

(c) Both (a) and (b)

(d) None of them

157. In eukaryotes, DNA is present inside the:

(a) Nucleus (b) Chloroplast

(c) Mitochondria (d) All of them

158. Stem cells are unspecialized cells that can:

(a) Replenish their number for long period

(b) Differentiate into specialized cells

(c) Both (a) and (b)

(d) None of them

159. Adult stem cell is undifferentiated cell, can:

(a) Differentiate to give specialized cells (b) Renew itself

(c) Both (a) and (b) (d) None of them

160. In a living animal, adult stem cell can divide for a long period and produce cell types having:

(a) Characteristic shapes
(b) Specialized structure
(c) Specialized function
(d) All of them

161. Diseases curable by stem cell therapy:

(a) Cystotic fibrosis
(b) Hutington's disease
(c) Spinal cord injuries
(d) All of them

162. Apoptosis plays essential role in the:

(a) Development of homeostasis
(b) Maintenance of homeostasis
(c) Host defence
(d) All of them

Answer Key

1	(c)	26	(d)	51	(a)	76	(d)
2	(a)	27	(b)	52	(a)	77	(d)
3	(b)	28	(d)	53	(a)	78	(d)
4	(c)	29	(a)	54	(c)	79	(c)
5	(b)	30	(a)	55	(a)	80	(c)
6	(d)	31	(d)	56	(a)	81	(d)
7	(c)	32	(a)	57	(d)	82	(d)
8	(c)	33	(d)	58	(c)	83	(a)
9	(a)	34	(a)	59	(c)	84	(a)
10	(a)	35	(d)	60	(d)	85	(d)
11	(c)	36	(a)	61	(d)	86	(c)
12	(a)	37	(a)	62	(d)	87	(c)
13	(a)	38	(d)	63	(c)	88	(d)
14	(b)	39	(d)	64	(d)	89	(c)
15	(a)	40	(c)	65	(c)	90	(c)
16	(b)	41	(d)	66	(c)	91	(b)
17	(a)	42	(d)	67	(a)	92	(d)
18	(d)	43	(c)	68	(c)	93	(c)
19	(a)	44	(d)	69	(d)	94	(a)
20	(a)	45	(a)	70	(c)	95	(c)
21	(b)	46	(a)	71	(d)	96	(c)
22	(c)	47	(a)	72	(c)	97	(d)
23	(a)	48	(c)	73	(a)	98	(b)
24	(a)	49	(a)	74	(d)	99	(b)
25	(c)	50	(a)	75	(a)	100	(d)

101	(d)	117	(c)	133	(d)	149	(c)
102	(a)	118	(c)	134	(d)	150	(d)
103	(a)	119	(d)	135	(c)	151	(d)
104	(a)	120	(c)	136	(c)	152	(c)
105	(a)	121	(c)	137	(d)	153	(d)
106	(a)	122	(c)	138	(c)	154	(c)
107	(d)	123	(c)	139	(d)	155	(d)
108	(d)	124	(c)	140	(d)	156	(c)
109	(c)	125	(d)	141	(d)	157	(d)
110	(d)	126	(c)	142	(d)	158	(c)
111	(c)	127	(c)	143	(d)	159	(c)
112	(c)	128	(d)	144	(c)	160	(d)
113	(c)	129	(d)	145	(d)	161	(d)
114	(c)	130	(d)	146	(d)	162	(d)
115	(d)	131	(c)	147	(c)		
116	(a)	132	(d)	148	(d)		

www.ingramcontent.com/pod-product-compliance
Ingram Content Group UK Ltd.
Pitfield, Milton Keynes, MK11 3LW, UK
UKHW021448280726
14060UKWH00001BA/305